DEMONSTRATING YOUR COMPETENCE 4: RESPIRATORY DISEASE, MENTAL HEALTH, DIABETES AND DERMATOLOGY

T0133909

Ruth Chambers
Gill Wakley
and
Alistair Pullan

RADCLIFFE PUBLISHING
Oxford • San Francisco

Radcliffe Publishing Ltd
18 Marcham Road
Abingdon
Oxon OX14 1AA
United Kingdom

www.radcliffe-oxford.com
Electronic catalogue and worldwide online ordering facility.

———————————————————————————

British Library Cataloguing in Publication Data

A catalogue record for this book is available from the British Library.

ISBN 1 85775 613 4

Typeset by Advance Typesetting Ltd, Oxford
Printed and bound by TJ International Ltd, Padstow, Cornwall

Contents

Preface

The General Medical Council has asked doctors to start thinking now about how they will collect and keep the information that will show that they should continue to hold a licence to practise as doctors from 2005 onwards. The onus will be on individual doctors to show that they are up to date and fit to practise medicine throughout their careers. It will be doctors who decide for themselves the nature of the information they collect and retain that best reflects their roles and responsibilities in their everyday work.

This book is one of a series that will guide you as a general practitioner though the process, giving you examples and ideas as to how to document your learning, competence, performance or standards of service delivery. At the same time as you are collecting the data to demonstrate your own competence, you are also helping to show that your practice is achieving high standards of care. The quality points available from the quality and outcomes framework of the General Medical Services (GMS) contract for general practice are achievable on a sliding scale.[1] As you increase your knowledge and skills in the clinical fields covered by the contract and improve your practice organisation with service developments, you should be working towards maximising your quality points. Some of the quality indicators are generic to various clinical areas such as smoking status, smoking cessation advice and influenza immunisation, and obviously overlap. Others such as good record keeping, consistent approach to maintaining disease registers, medicines management and education/appraisal of staff should underpin all the clinical areas. As we cover the seven clinical topics in this book in Chapters 4 to 10, we point out what quality points are available in that clinical area. Other books in the series also include clinical topics within the scope of the GMS contract – so it will be useful for you to read them too (e.g. coronary heart disease and stroke are included in: Wakley G, Chambers R and Ellis S (2004) *Demonstrating Your Competence 3: Cardiovascular and Neurological Conditions.* Radcliffe Publishing, Oxford).

Chapter 1 explains the link between your personal development plans, local appraisal and the revalidation of your medical registration. Learning and service improvements that are integral to your personal development plan are central to the evidence you include in your appraisal and revalidation portfolio.

The stages of the evidence cycle that we suggest are built upon the underpinning publication: Chambers R, Wakley G, Field S and Ellis S (2003) *Appraisal for the Apprehensive.* Radcliffe Medical Press, Oxford.

Stage 1 is about setting targets or aspirations for good practice. Many of the aspirations we suggest are taken from *Good Medical Practice*[2] or its sister publication, *Good Medical Practice for General Practitioners*.[3] Stage 2 encourages you, as a doctor, to set standards for the outcomes of what you plan to learn more about, or outcomes relating to you providing a good service in your practice.

Chapter 2 describes a variety of methods to help you to address Stage 3 of the cycle of evidence, to find out what it is you need to learn about or what gaps there are in the way you deliver care as an individual general practitioner (GP) or as a team. This chapter includes a wide variety of methods doctors might use in their everyday work to identify and document these needs. One of the drivers for the introduction of appraisal and revalidation has been to reassure the public and others of doctors' continuing fitness to practise. So it makes sense that we have emphasised the importance of obtaining feedback from patients in this chapter in relation to identifying your learning and service development needs.

Best practice in addressing the giving of informed consent by patients, maintaining confidentiality of patient information and organising responsive complaints processes are all common components of good quality healthcare. Chapter 3 covers these aspects in depth and provides the first example of cycles of evidence for you to consider adopting or adapting for your own circumstances. The focus of each cycle of evidence is on one of the 'headings' from *Good Medical Practice*[2] or standard appraisal format.

The rest of the book consists of seven clinically based chapters that span key topics in chronic disease. The first part of each chapter covers key issues that are likely to crop up in typical consultations for each clinical field. The second part of each chapter gives examples of cycles of evidence in a similar format to those in Chapter 3.

Overall, you will probably want to choose three or four cycles of evidence each year. You might choose one or two cycles from Chapter 3 and the rest from clinical areas such as those covered by Chapters 4 to 10. You might like this way of learning and service development so much that you build up a bigger bank of evidence, taking one cycle from each chapter in the same year. Whatever your approach, you will want to keep your cycles of evidence as short and simple as possible, so that the documentation itself is a by-product of the learning and action plans you undertake to improve the service you provide, and does not dominate your time and effort at work.

Other books in the series are based on the same format of the five stages in the cycle of evidence. Book 1 helps doctors and other health professionals to demonstrate that they are competent teachers or trainers, and Books 2, 3 and 5 set out key information and examples of evidence for a wide variety of clinical areas for GPs and other doctors.

This approach and style of learning will take a bit of getting used to for doctors. Until now, they have not had to prove that they are fit to practise unless the General Medical Council has investigated them for a significant reason such as a complaint or error. Until recently, most doctors did not evaluate what they learnt or whether they applied it in practice. They did not protect time for learning and reflection among their everyday responsibilities, or target their time and effort on priority topics. Times are changing, and with the introduction of personal development plans and appraisal, GPs are realising that they must take a more professional approach to learning and document their standards of competence, performance and service delivery. This book helps them to do just that.

Please note that resources to support this book are provided at http://health.mattersonline.net

References

1 General Practitioners Committee/The NHS Confederation (2003) *New GMS Contract. Investing in general practice.* General Practitioners Committee/NHS Confederation, London.

2 General Medical Council (2001) *Good Medical Practice.* General Medical Council, London.

3 Royal College of General Practitioners/General Practitioners Committee (2002) *Good Medical Practice for General Practitioners.* Royal College of General Practitioners, London.

About the authors

Ruth Chambers has been a GP for more than 20 years and is currently the head of the Stoke-on-Trent Teaching Primary Care Trust programme and professor of primary care development at Staffordshire University. Ruth has worked with the Royal College of General Practitioners to enable GPs to gather evidence about their learning and standards of practice while striving to be excellent GPs. Ruth has co-authored a series of books with Gill, designed to help readers draw up their own personal development plans or workplace learning plans around key clinical topics.

Gill Wakley started in general practice but transferred to community medicine shortly afterwards and then into public health. A desire for increased contact with patients caused a move back into general practice. She has been heavily involved in learning and teaching throughout her career. She was in a training general practice, became an instructing doctor and a regional assessor in family planning, and was until recently a senior clinical lecturer with the Primary Care Department at Keele University. Like Ruth, she has run all types of educational initiatives and activities. A visiting professor at Staffordshire University, she now works as a freelance GP, writer and lecturer.

Alistair Pullan graduated from Aberdeen University in 1985. Having completed his pre-registration house jobs in Aberdeen and Inverness, he moved to England, completing the North Staffordshire General Practitioner Vocational Training Scheme in 1990. Since then he has worked as a full-time principal in general practice in Stoke-on-Trent. He was awarded the Diploma in Practical Dermatology by the University of Wales College of Medicine in 2001. In addition to his work as a GP, Alistair is a GP with special interest in dermatology.

1

Making the link: personal development plans, appraisal and revalidation

The nexus of personal development plans, appraisal and revalidation

Learning involves many steps. It includes the acquisition of information, its retention, the ability to retrieve the information when needed and how to use that information for best practice. Demonstrating your learning involves being able to show the steps you have taken. Learning should be lifelong and encompass continuing professional development.

Continuing professional development (CPD) takes time. It makes sense to utilise the time spent by overlapping learning to meet your personal and professional needs with that required for the performance of your role in the health service.

Many doctors have drawn up a personal development plan (PDP) that is agreed with their local CPD or college tutor. Some doctors have constructed their PDP in a systematic way and identified the priorities within it, or gathered evidence to demonstrate that what they learnt about was subsequently applied in practice. Tutors do not have a uniform approach to the style and relevance of a doctor's PDP. Some are content that a plan has been drawn up, while others encourage the doctor to develop a systematic approach to identifying and addressing their learning and service needs, in order of importance or urgency.[1]

The new emphasis on doctors' accountability to the public has given the PDP a higher profile and shown that it may be used in other ways. The medical education establishment and NHS management argue about the balance between its alternative uses. The educationalists view a PDP as a tool to encourage doctors to plan their own learning activities. The management view is of a tool allowing quality assurance of the doctor's performance. Doctors, striving to improve the quality of the care that they deliver to patients, want to use a PDP to guide them on their way, perhaps towards postgraduate awards of universities or the quality awards of the Royal College of General Practitioners. These quality awards are built around the standards of excellence to which a GP should aspire, as described in the publication, *Good Medical Practice for General Practitioners.*[2]

Your personal development plan

Your PDP will be an integral part of your future appraisal and revalidation portfolio to demonstrate your fitness to practise as a doctor.

Your initial plan should:

- identify your gaps or weaknesses in knowledge, skills or attitudes
- specify topics for learning as a result of changes: in your role, responsibilities, the organisation in which you work
- link into the learning needs of others in your workplace or team of colleagues
- tie in with the service development priorities of your practice, the primary care organisation (PCO) or the NHS as a whole
- describe how you identified your learning needs
- set your learning needs and associated goals in order of importance and urgency
- justify your selection of learning goals
- describe how you will achieve your goals and over what time period
- describe how you will evaluate learning outcomes.

Each year you will continue or revise your PDP. It should demonstrate how you carried out your learning and evaluation plans, show that you have learnt what you set out to do (or why it was modified) and how you applied your new learning in practice. In addition, you will find that you have new priorities and fresh learning needs as circumstances change.

The main task is to capture what you have learnt, in a way that suits you. Then you can look back at what you have done and:

- reflect on it later, to decide to learn more, or to make changes as a result, and identify further needs
- demonstrate to others that you are fit to practise or work through:
  - what you have done
  - what you have learnt
  - what changes you have made as a result
  - the standards of work you have achieved and are maintaining
  - how you monitor your performance at work
- use it to show how your personal learning fits in with the requirements of your practice or the NHS, and other people's personal and professional development plans.

Organise all the evidence of your learning into a CPD portfolio of some sort. It is up to you how you keep this record of your learning. Examples are:

- *an ongoing learning journal* in which you draw up and describe your plan, record how you determined your needs and prioritised them, report why you attended particular educational meetings or courses and what you got out of them as well as the continuing cycle of review, making changes and evaluating them
- *an A4 file* with lots of plastic sleeves into which you build up a systematic record of your educational activities in line with your plan
- *a box*: chuck in everything to do with your learning plan as you do it and sort it out into a sensible order every few months with a good review once a year.

The context of appraisal and revalidation

Appraisal and revalidation are based on the same sources of information – presented in the same structure as the headings set out in the General Medical Council (GMC) guidance in *Good Medical Practice*.[3] The two processes perform different functions. Whereas revalidation involves an assessment against a standard of fitness to practise medicine, appraisal is concerned with the doctor's professional development within his or her working environment and the needs of the organisation for which the doctor works.

Appraisal is a formative and developmental process that is being introduced by the Departments of Health for all general practitioners (GPs) and hospital consultants working in the NHS across the UK. While the details of the appraisal system vary for consultants and GPs and for each of the countries, the educational principles remain the same. The aims of the appraisal system are to give doctors an opportunity to discuss and receive regular feedback on their previous and continuing performance and identify education and development needs.

The drive to introduce formal appraisals came initially as part of the programme to introduce clinical governance across the NHS as laid out in the 1998 consultation document *A First Class Service*.[4] Momentum was gained with the publication of *Supporting Doctors, Protecting Patients* (1999) in England which outlined a set of proposals to help prevent doctors from developing problems.[5] Appraisal was at the heart of the proposals as:

a positive process to give someone feedback on their performance, to chart their continuing progress and to identify development needs. It is a forward looking process essential for the developmental and educational planning needs of an individual. *Assessment* is the process of measuring progress against agreed criteria . . . . It is not the primary aim of appraisal to scrutinise doctors to see if they are performing poorly but rather to help them consolidate and improve on good performance aiming towards excellence.[5]

The document went on to suggest that appraisal should be made comprehensive and compulsory for doctors working in the NHS and form part of a future revalidation system.

In addition, appraisal should also address other areas of particular importance to the individual doctor. A standardised approach has been developed that utilises approved documentation. This should ensure that information from a variety of NHS employers is recorded consistently. The format of the paperwork is slightly different for consultants and GPs.

Appraisal must be a positive, formative and developmental process to support high quality patient care and improve clinical standards. Appraisal is different from, but linked to, revalidation.[6] Revalidation is the process whereby doctors will be regularly required to demonstrate that they are fit to practise. Appraisal feeds into this by contributing to the information that a doctor supplies for the revalidation process. Appraisal will provide a regular structured recording system for documenting progress towards revalidation and identifying needs as part of the doctor's PDPs. Both the NHS appraisal and the revalidation structures are based on the same seven headings set out in the GMC's guidance *Good Medical Practice*.[3] The GMC claims, therefore, that 'five satisfactory appraisals equals revalidation'.[6] The GMC has also pledged that doctors not taking part in appraisal will be able to provide their own information for revalidation, providing this evidence meets the same criteria as in *Good Medical Practice.*

Appraisal is, however, a two-way process. Not only time, but also resources will be needed to make appraisal systems successful. In addition, appraisal will identify issues that will require extra investment by the NHS in the educational and organisational infrastructure.

Appraisal and revalidation processes are being increasingly integrated. The PDP is a central part of the appraisal documentation, which will in turn be included in the portfolio of information available for revalidation. It seems that the evolution will continue so that revalidation is met by supporting the appraisal documentation with additional documents about clinical governance activity and CPD. These supporting documents will be a mix of subjective and objective information that will include doctors' self-assessment of their performance and other work-based assessment.

The revalidation and appraisal processes need to be quality assured to be able to demonstrate that they can protect the public from poor or underperforming doctors. Such quality assurance will relate to the appraisers, their training and support, as well as systems to examine the quality of evidence in the documentation relating to a doctor's performance and outcomes of their PDP. You should regard your PDP and supporting documentation as central to the way in which you can show, to anyone who requires you to do so, that your performance as a doctor is acceptable and that you are trying to improve, or striving for excellence.

Demonstrating the standards of your practice

The GMC sets out standards that must be met as part of the duties and responsibilities of doctors in the booklet *Good Medical Practice*.[3] Doctors must be able to meet these standards with a record of their own performance in their revalidation portfolio if they want to retain a licence to practise. The nine key headings of expected standards of practice for all general practitioners working in England are shown in Box 1.1.

Box 1.1:   Key headings of expected standards of practice for GPs working in England

1 *Good professional practice.* This relates to clinical care, keeping records (including writing reports and keeping colleagues informed), access and availability, treatment in emergencies and making effective use of resources.
2 *Maintaining good medical practice.* This includes keeping up to date and maintaining your performance.
3 *Relationships with patients.* This encompasses providing information about your services, maintaining trust, avoiding discrimination and prejudice against patients, relating well to patients and apologising if things go wrong.
4 *Working with colleagues.* This relates to working with colleagues, working in teams, referring patients and accepting posts.
5 *Teaching and training, appraising and assessing.* You may be in a position to teach or train colleagues or students, and appraise or assess peers, employees or students.
6 *Probity* includes providing true information about your services, honesty in financial and commercial dealings, and providing references.
7 *Health* can include how you overcome or compensate for health problems in yourself, or help with or address health problems in other doctors.
8 *Research.* Conducting research in an ethical manner.
9 *Management.* The section on management concerns any responsibility GPs have for management outside the practice. GPs might wish to include management responsibilities that cross the interface between their practice and PCO.

The appraisal paperwork for GPs working in England, Scotland, Wales and Northern Ireland has been individualised by each country. The English version, for example, includes two extra sections to those of hospital consultants – management and research. The Scottish version focuses on core categories in preparation for revalidation of prescribing, referrals and peer review, clinical audit, significant event analysis and communication skills, summary of any complaints and other feedback.

The stages of the evidence cycle for demonstrating your standards of practice or competence and any necessary improvements are given in Figure 1.1. The stages of the evidence cycle are common to all the various areas of expertise considered in this book and will be followed in each chapter.

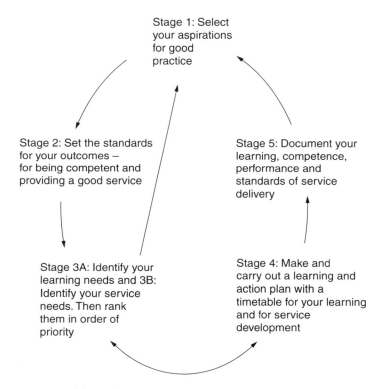

Figure 1.1:   Stages of the evidence cycle.

Although the five stages are shown in sequence here, in practice you would expect to move backwards and forwards from stage to stage, because of new information or a modification of your earlier ideas. New information might accrue when research is published which affects your clinical behaviour or standards, or a critical incident or patient complaint might occur which causes you and others to think anew about your standards or the way that services are delivered. The arrows in Figure 1.1 show that you might re-set your target or aspirations for good practice having undertaken exercises to identify what you need to learn or determine whether there are gaps in service delivery.

We suggest that you demonstrate your competence in focused areas of your day-to-day work by completing several cycles of evidence drawn from a variety of clinical or other areas each year, with at least one cycle of evidence from each of the main headings of *Good Medical Practice* over a five-year cycle.[3] By demonstrating your standards of practice around the main sections of *Good Medical Practice*, you will document your competence and performance for your revalidation portfolio in the same format as that required for your appraisal paperwork.

As you start to collate information about this five-stage cycle, discuss any problems about the standards of care or services you are looking at, with colleagues, experts in this area, tutors, etc. You want to develop a wide range and depth of evidence so that you can show that you are competent in your day-to-day general work as well as for any special areas of expertise.

Professional competence is the first area of concern in *Good Medical Practice*.[3] You should be able to demonstrate that you can maintain a satisfactory standard of clinical care most of the time in your everyday work. Some of the time you will be brilliant, of course! Celebrate those moments. On other occasions, you or others will be critical of your performance and feel that you could have done much better. Reflect on those episodes to learn from them.

Stage 1: Select your aspirations for good practice

By adopting or adapting descriptions of what an 'excellent' GP should be aiming for, you are defining the standards of practice for which all doctors should be aiming. The medical Royal Colleges have interpreted *Good Medical Practice* in various ways for the specialities of their own members.[3] For example, *Good Medical Practice for General Practitioners* describes the standards of practice that should be achieved by 'excellent' or 'unacceptable' GPs.[2] Their definition of excellence is being 'consistently good'.

This consistency is a critical factor in considering competence and perform-ance too (*see* page 16). The documents that you collect in your evidence cycles must reflect consistency over time and in different circumstances, for example with various types of patients or your practice at different times of day. This will show that you have not only performed well on one occasion or for one type of baseline assessment, but also sustained your performance over time and under different conditions.

Stage 2: Set the standards for your outcomes – for being competent and providing a good service

Outcomes might include:

- the way that learning is applied
- a learnt skill
- a protocol
- a strategy that is implemented
- meeting recommended standards.

The level at which you should be performing depends on your particular field of expertise. GPs are good at seeing the wider picture, while specialists tend to be expert in a narrow area, so that the level of competence expected for a clinical area will vary depending on the doctor's role and responsibilities. You would not, for example, expect orthopaedic specialists to be competent at managing cardiac failure (although some of them may be), but you would expect GPs be able to manage all but the most complicated situations involving cardiac failure. You would expect both the orthopaedic specialist and the GP to recognise the limits of their competence and to refer to someone with more expertise when necessary.

Other standards include using resources effectively and the record keeping that is an essential tool in clinical care. As a health professional, you need to be accessible and available so that you can provide your services, and make suitable arrangements for handing over care to others. You must provide care in an emergency.

You could incorporate into your standards or outcomes those components specified by universities at a national level as part of their Masters' Frameworks for their postgraduate awards. The Masters' Frameworks consist of eight components that shape the individual postgraduate award programme outcomes and the learning outcomes of the individual modules for the postgraduate awards. The eight components are shown in Box 1.2. You could set out your CPD work in the portfolio you are assembling for revalidation and your annual appraisals in this format. This would help you to document your professional development to date in a form that can be readily 'accredited for prior experiential learning' (APEL) by universities (contact your local universities if you want more information about this process). You might then be given credits for learning against an intended postgraduate award. It would save you from duplicating work as well as speeding your progress through the award.

Box 1.2: The eight components of the Masters' Frameworks for postgraduate awards

1 Analysis
2 Problem solving
3 Knowledge and understanding
4 Reflection
5 Communication
6 Learning
7 Application
8 Enquiry

If you have information or data about your practice showing that it was substandard or that you were not competent, you might choose to exclude that from your portfolio. However, you will be able to show that you have learnt more by reviewing mistakes or negative episodes. It is better to include everything of relevance, then go on to demonstrate how you addressed the gaps in your performance and made sustained improvements. You will need to protect the confidentiality of patients and colleagues as necessary when you collect data. The GMC will be seeing the contents of your revalidation portfolio if your submission is one of those sampled. You will probably also submit or share the documentation for appraisal and maybe use it for reviews with colleagues or the PCO.

Stage 3: Identify your learning and service needs in your practice or primary care organisation and rank them in order of priority[1]

The type and depth of documentation you need to gather will encompass:

• the context in which you work
• your knowledge and skills in relation to any particular role or responsibility of your current post.

The extent of expertise you should possess will depend on your level of responsibility for a particular function or task. You may be personally responsible for that function or task, or you may contribute or delegate responsibility for it. Your learning needs should take into account your aspirations for the future too – personal or career development for you, or improvements in the way you deliver care in your practice. Look at Chapter 2 for more ideas on how you will identify your learning or service development needs.

Group and summarise your service development needs from the exercises you have carried out. Grade them according to the priority you set. You may put one at a higher priority because it fits in with service development needs established in the business plan of the trust or practice, or put another lower because it does not fit in with other activities that your organisation has in their current development plan for the next 12 months. If you have identified a service development need by several different methods of assessment or with several different patient groups or clinical conditions, then it will have a higher priority than something only identified once. Notify the service development needs you have identified to those responsible for agreeing and implementing the development plans of the trust and/or practice.

Look back at your aspirations and standards set out in Stages 1 and 2. Match your learning or service development needs with one or more of these standards, or others that you have set yourself.

Stage 4: Make and carry out a learning and action plan with a timetable for your personal and service development

If you have not identified any learning needs for yourself or the service as a whole, you should omit Stage 4 and tidy up the presentation of your evidence for inclusion in your portfolio as at the end of Stage 5.

Think about whether:

- you have defined your learning objectives – what you need to learn to be able to attain the standards and outcomes you have described in Stage 2
- you can justify spending time and effort on the topics you prioritised in Stage 3. Is the topic important enough to your work, the NHS as a whole or patient safety? Does the clinical or non-clinical event occur sufficiently often to warrant the time spent?
- the time and resources for learning about that topic or making the associated changes to service delivery are available. Check that you are not trying to do too much too quickly, or you will become discouraged
- learning about that topic will make a difference to the care you or others can provide for patients
- and how one topic fits in with other topics you have identified to learn more about. Have you achieved a good balance across your areas of work or between your personal aspirations and the basic requirements of the service?

Decide on what method of learning is most appropriate for your task or role or the standards you are expecting to attain or sustain. You may have already identified your preferred learning style – but read up on this elsewhere if you are unsure.[7]

Describe how you will carry out your learning tasks and what you will do by a specified time. State how your learning will be applied and how and when it will be evaluated. Build in some staging posts so that you do not suddenly get to the end of 12 months and discover that you have only done half of your plan.

Your action plan should also include your role in remedying any gaps in service delivery that you identified in Stage 3 that are within the remit of your responsibility.

Stage 5: Document your learning, competence, performance and standards of service delivery

You might choose to document that you have attained your defined outcomes by repeating the learning needs assessment that you started with. You could record your increased confidence and competence in dealing with situations that you previously avoided or performed inadequately.

You might incorporate your assessment of what has been gained in a study of another area that overlaps.

Preparing your portfolio[8-10]

Use your portfolio of evidence of what you have learnt and your standards of practice to:

- identify significant experiences to serve as important sources of learning
- reflect on the learning that arose from those experiences
- demonstrate learning in practice
- analyse and identify further learning needs and ways in which these needs can be met.

Your documentation might include all sorts of things, not just formal audits – although they make a good start. It might include reports of educational activities attended, statements of your roles and responsibilities, copies of publications you have read and critically appraised, and reports of your work. You could incorporate observations by others, evaluations of yourself observing other colleagues and how their practice differs from yours, descriptions of self-improvements, a video of typical activity, materials that demonstrate your skills to others, products of your input or learning – a new protocol for example. Box 1.3 gives a list of material you might include in your portfolio.

Box 1.3:   Possible contents of a portfolio

- Workload logs
- Case descriptions
- Videos
- Audiotapes
- Patient satisfaction surveys
- Research surveys
- Report of change or innovation
- Commentaries on published literature or books
- Records of critical incidents and learning points
- Notes from formal teaching sessions with reference to clinical work or other evidence

---

Once you are preparing to submit the portfolio for a discussion with a colleague (for example, at an appraisal) or assessment (for example, for a university postgraduate award or revalidation), write a self-assessment of your previous action plan. You might integrate your self-assessment into your PDP to show what you have achieved and what gaps you have still to address. Decide where you are now and where you want to be in one, three or five years' time. Select items from your portfolio for inclusion for each part of the documentation – you might have one compartment of your portfolio per speciality topic or section heading from *Good Medical Practice*.[3]

Make sure all references are included and the documentation in your portfolio is as accurate and complete as possible. Organise how you have shown your learning steps and your standards of practice so that it is indexed and cross-referenced to the relevant sections of the paperwork. Discuss the contents of your portfolio with a colleague or a mentor to gain other people's perspectives of your work and look for blind spots.

Include evidence of your competence as a GP with a special interest (GPwSI)

You may have a particular expertise or special interest in a clinical field or non-clinical area such as management, teaching or research. It may be that you have a lead role or responsibility in your practice for chronic disease management of clinical conditions such as diabetes, asthma, mental health or coronary heart disease. Or you may be employed by a PCO or hospital trust as a GPwSI to:

- lead in the development of services
- deliver a procedure-based service
- deliver an opinion-based service.

There is little consistency in extent of training or qualifications at present within or across the various GPwSI specialty areas.[11] Whatever your role, responsibility or expertise, your portfolio should include examples of evidence that show that you are competent, and that you have a consistently good performance in your specialty area. You may have parallel appraisals that you can include from your employer – for example, the university if you have a research or teaching post, or a hospital consultant if he or she supervises you in the clinical specialty.

When you gather evidence of your performance at work, try to document as many aspects of your work at one time as you can, so that for example an audit covers as many of the key headings from *Good Medical Practice* (*see* Box 1.1 page 5) as possible.[3] When you are identifying what you need to learn, or gaps in service delivery, make sure that you involve patients and show how you interact with the team. This gives you evidence about 'relationships with patients' and 'working with colleagues' as well as the clinical area you are focusing on or auditing.

Link your cycles of evidence to service developments rewarded by the new General Medical Services (GMS) Contract or Personal Medical Services (PMS) arrangements

The areas within the quality framework will probably be the ones that you prioritise in your PDP when looking at your service development needs.[12] The four main components of the quality framework are all relevant to your personal and professional development. The clinical and organisational standards may be those which you are aiming for in Stage 2 of the evidence cycle (*see* Figure 1.1). Achieving the standards in the quality framework will follow on from the descriptions of an excellent GP (Stage 1). Identifying personal learning needs and service development needs, that is, the gaps between baseline and specified standards in the quality framework, is in Stage 3. Making and carrying out your personal learning plan and service improvements in line with patients' experience is in Stage 4. Producing the documentation that shows you have attained the clinical or organisational standards required for core or additional services and responded to patients' views is in Stage 5.

References

1   Wakley G, Chambers R and Field S (2000) *Continuing Professional Development in Primary Care.* Radcliffe Medical Press, Oxford.

2   Royal College of General Practitioners/General Practitioners Committee (2002) *Good Medical Practice for General Practitioners.* Royal College of General Practitioners, London.

3   General Medical Council (2001) *Good Medical Practice.* General Medical Council, London.

4   Department of Health (1998) *A First Class Service.* Department of Health, London.

5   Department of Health (1999) *Supporting Doctors, Protecting Patients.* Department of Health, London.

6   General Medical Council (2003) *Licence to Practise and Revalidation for Doctors.* General Medical Council, London. www.revalidationuk.info

7   Mohanna K, Wall D and Chambers R (2003) *Teaching Made Easy: a manual for health professionals* (2e). Radcliffe Medical Press, Oxford.

8   Royal College of General Practitioners (1993) *Portfolio-based Learning in General Practice.* Occasional Paper 63, Royal College of General Practitioners, London.

9   Challis M (1999) AMEE Medical education guide No 11 (revised): portfolio-based learning and assessment in medical education. *Medical Teacher.* **21(4):** 370–86.

10   Chambers C, Wakley G, Field S and Ellis S (2003) *Appraisal for the Apprehensive.* Radcliffe Medical Press, Oxford.

11   www.gpwsi.org

12   General Practitioners Committee/The NHS Confederation (2003) *New GMS Contract. Investing in general practice.* General Practitioners Committee/NHS Confederation, London.

2

Practical ways to identify your learning and service needs as part of the documentation of your competence and performance

Setting standards to show that you are competent

> Doctors 'must be committed to lifelong learning and be responsible for maintaining the medical knowledge and clinical and team skills necessary for the provision of quality care'.[1]

You could make a good start by describing your roles and responsibilities. This will help you to define what your competence should be now, or what competence you are hoping to attain (for instance as a GPwSI). Once you have your definition, you can recognise whether you have, or lack in some part, the necessary competence. If there are no accepted descriptions of competence in the area you are focusing on, then you will have to start from scratch. You might compile your description from national guidelines such as in the National Service Frameworks or health strategies. Usually you can find guidance about competency from specialist sources such as primary care associations for clinical topics or the various Royal Colleges. The Department of Health in England has worked with the Royal College of General Practitioners (RCGP) to describe the competency of GPs with special clinical interests in many clinical areas.[2]

A good definition of competence is someone who is: 'able to perform the tasks and roles required to the expected standard'.[3]

You will need to describe the standards expected in the range of tasks and roles you undertake and reference the source of standard setting. If professionals, or their organisations, are the only people involved in setting those standards, consider whether you should amend or extend the standards, tasks or roles by considering other perspectives such as those of patients or the NHS as a whole.

There is a difference between being competent, and performing in a consistently competent manner. You need to be motivated to perform consistently well and enabled to do so with efficient systems and sufficient resources. You will require sufficient numbers of other competent doctors or staff and available infrastructure such as diagnostic and treatment resources.[4]

Choose methods in Stage 3 (*see* Chapter 1) to demonstrate your standards of performance and identify any learning needs that span different topic areas, to reduce duplication and maximise the usefulness of your learning. Collecting evidence of more than one aspect of your competence or performance cuts down the overall amount of work underpinning your PDP or included in your appraisal portfolio.

Use several methods to identify your learning needs and/or gaps in your service development or delivery, so that you validate the findings of one method by another. No one method will give you reliable information about the gaps in your knowledge, skills or attitudes or everyday service. Does what you think about your performance match with what others in the team or patients think of how you practise in your everyday work? It is particularly difficult to determine what it is you 'don't know you don't know' by yourself, yet it is vital that you identify and rectify those gaps. Other people may be able to tell you what you need to learn quite readily. Colleagues from different disciplines could usefully comment on any shortfalls in how your work interfaces with theirs.

Patients or people who don't use your services could tell you whether the way you operate or provide services is off-putting or inappropriate. There may be data about your performance or that of your practice that could point out those gaps in your knowledge or skills of which you were previously unaware.

Determine what it is that you 'don't know you don't know' by:

- asking patients, users and non-users of your service
- comparing your performance against best practice or that of peers
- comparing your performance against objectives in business plans or national directives
- asking colleagues from different disciplines about shortfalls in how your work interfaces with theirs.

Identify your learning needs – how you can find out if you need to be better at doing your job

You may decide to use a few selected methods to gather baseline evidence of your performance, focused on your specific area of expertise. You may target other topics or areas at the same time that are relevant to the various sections of the GMC's booklet *Good Medical Practice*.[5] For this type of combined assessment, you might use several of the methods described in this chapter such as:

- constructive feedback from peers or patients
- 360° feedback
- self-assessment, or review by others, using a rating scale to assess your skills and attitudes
- comparison with protocols and guidelines for checking how well procedures are followed
- audit: various types and applications
- significant event audit
- eliciting patient views such as satisfaction surveys
- a SWOT (strengths, weaknesses, opportunities and threats) or SCOT (strengths, challenges, opportunities and threats) analysis
- reading and reflecting
- educational review.

Several of these methods will also be useful for identifying service development needs – you can look at the gaps identified from both the personal and service perspectives at the same time using the same method.

Seek feedback

Find colleagues who will give you constructive feedback about your performance and practice. The golden rule for giving constructive feedback is to give positive praise of things that have been well done first. Sometimes colleagues launch straight in to criticise faults when asked for their views. The Pendleton model of the giving of feedback is widely used in the health setting (*see* Box 2.1).[6]

Box 2.1:
The Pendleton model of giving feedback

1 The 'learner' goes first and performs the activity.
2 The teacher questions or clarifies any facts.
3 The 'learner' says what they thought was done well.
4 The 'teacher' says what they thought was done well.
5 The 'learner' says what could be improved upon.
6 The 'teacher' says what could be improved upon.
7 Both discuss ideas for improvements in a helpful and constructive manner.

360° feedback

This collects together perceptions from a number of different participants as shown in Figure 2.1.

People to whom you are responsible: managers in your PCO, appraiser, clinical lead, clinical governance lead, GP partners etc

Your peers or colleagues ——————► **You** ◄—————— Patients or carers

People responsible to you: clinical and non-clinical staff

Figure 2.1:   360° feedback.

The wider the spread of people giving feedback, the more rounded the picture. Each individual gives a feedback questionnaire to at least three people in each of the groups above. An independent person then collects and collates the questionnaires and discusses the results with the individual. Computerised versions are available from commercial companies.[7] The main disadvantage of this method is that it can sometimes be spoilt by malicious comments against which individuals cannot readily defend themselves.

Self-assess or gain another person's perspective on your standard of practice or service delivery

You might describe any aspect of your practice as statements (A to G as in Box 2.2) about your competence or performance for you to self-assess or others to give you feedback or comments by marking the extent to which they agree on the linear scales below. You could use the descriptions of an excellent GP in

---

Box 2.2: Marking grid: circle the number which represents your views or feelings about each statement – complete the grid on more than one occasion and compare results over time

A I consistently treat patients politely and with consideration.

STRONGLY AGREE   to   STRONGLY DISAGREE

1----------------2----------------3----------------4----------------5----------------6

B I am aware of how my personal beliefs could affect the care offered to the patient, and take care not to impose my own beliefs and values.

STRONGLY AGREE   to   STRONGLY DISAGREE

1----------------2----------------3----------------4----------------5----------------6

C I always treat all patients equally and ensure that some groups are not favoured at the expense of others.

STRONGLY AGREE   to   STRONGLY DISAGREE

1----------------2----------------3----------------4----------------5----------------6

D I try to maintain a relationship with the patient or family when a mistake has occurred.

STRONGLY AGREE   to   STRONGLY DISAGREE

1----------------2----------------3----------------4----------------5----------------6

E I always obtain informed consent to treatment.

STRONGLY AGREE   to   STRONGLY DISAGREE

1----------------2----------------3----------------4----------------5----------------6

F I usually involve patients in decisions about their care.

STRONGLY AGREE   to   STRONGLY DISAGREE

1----------------2----------------3----------------4----------------5----------------6

G I always respect the right of patients to refuse treatments or tests.

STRONGLY AGREE   to   STRONGLY DISAGREE

1----------------2----------------3----------------4----------------5----------------6

Good Medical Practice for General Practitioners[8] as we have done in relating statements in Box 2.2 to consultation skills. For instance, if statement A is: 'I consistently treat patients politely and with consideration',[8] you could self-assess the extent to which you agree. Alternatively, you could ask colleagues or patients to fill in the assessment form. Objective feedback from external assessment is usually more reliable than your own self-assessment when you may have blind spots about your own performance. As you become more confident in this method of reviewing your competence, you might emphasise how consistent you are in your application of good practice – so in the statements we have sometimes included 'consistently', 'always' or 'usually'. You can set your own challenges. If you have a mentor or a 'buddy' in the practice with whom you learn, you might discuss and reflect on the completed marking grids with him or her.

Compare your performance against protocols or guidelines

Are you familiar with all the protocols or guidelines that are used by someone, somewhere in the practice? You might determine your learning needs and those of other practice team members by piling all the protocols or guidelines that exist in your practice in a big heap and rationalising them so that you have a common set across the practice. Working as a team you can compare your own knowledge and usual practice with others and with protocols or guidelines recommended by the National Institute for Clinical Excellence (NICE)[9] or National Service Frameworks or the Scottish Intercollegiate Guidelines Network (SIGN).[10]

Alternatively, you might compare your own practice against a protocol or guideline that is generally accepted at a national or local level. You could audit the standard of your practice to find out how often you adhere to such a protocol or guideline, and if you can justify why you deviate from the recommendations.

Audit

Audit is:

> the method used by health professionals to assess, evaluate, and improve the care of patients in a systematic way, to enhance their health and quality of life.[11]

The five steps of the audit cycle are shown in Box 2.3.

Box 2.3: The five steps of the audit cycle

1 Describe the criteria and standards you are trying to achieve.
2 Measure your current performance of how well you are providing care or services in an objective way.
3 Compare your performance against criteria and standards.
4 Identify the need for change – to performance, adjustment of criteria or standards, resources, available data.
5 Make any required changes as necessary and re-audit later.

Performance or practice is often broken down for the purposes of audit into the three aspects of structure, process and outcome. Structural audits might concern resources such as equipment, premises, skills, people, etc. Process audits focus on what is done to the patient: for instance, clinical protocols and guidelines. Audits of outcomes consider the impact of care or services on the patient and might include patient satisfaction, health gains and effectiveness of care or services. You might look at aspects of quality of the structure, process and outcome of the delivery of any clinical field – focusing on access, equity of care between different groups in the population, efficiency, economy, effectiveness for individual patients, etc.[11]

Set standards for your performance, find out how you are doing, search to find out best practice, make the changes and then re-audit the care given to patients in the future with the same problem. Some variations on audit include:

- *Case note analysis.* This gives an insight into your current practice. It might be a retrospective review of a random selection of notes, or a prospective survey of consecutive patients with the same condition as they present to see you.
- *Peer review.* Compare an area of practice with other individual professionals or managers; or compare practice teams as a whole. An independent body might compare all practices in one area e.g. within a primary care organisation (PCO) so that like is compared with like. Feedback may be arranged to protect participants' identities so that only the individual person or practice knows their own identity, the rest being anonymised, for example by giving each practice a number. Where there is mutual trust and an open learning culture, peer review does not need to be anonymised and everyone can learn together about making improvements in practice.

- *Criteria-based audit*. This compares clinical practice with specific standards, guidelines or protocols. Re-audit of changes should demonstrate improvements in the quality of patient care.
- *External audit*. Prescribing advisers or managers in PCOs can supply information about indicators of performance for audit. Visits from external bodies such as the Healthcare Commission expose the PCO or hospital trust in England and Wales to external audit.
- *Tracer criteria*. Assessing the quality of care of a 'tracer' condition may be used to represent the quality of care of other similar conditions or more complex problems. Tracer criteria should be easily defined and measured. For instance, if you were to audit the extent to which you reviewed repeat prescriptions, you might focus on a drug such as thyroxine and generalise from your audit results to your likely performance with other medications.

Significant event audit

Think of an incident where a patient or you experienced an adverse event. This might be an unexpected death, an unplanned pregnancy, an avoidable side-effect from prescribed medication, a violent attack on a member of staff, or an angry outburst in public by you or a work colleague. You can review the case and reflect on the sequence of events that led to that critical event occurring. It is likely that there were a multitude of factors leading up to that significant event. You should take the case to a multidisciplinary meeting to reflect and analyse what were the triggers, causes and consequences of the event. Complete the significant event audit cycle by planning what individuals or the practice as a whole might do to avoid a similar event happening in future. This might include undertaking further learning and/or making appropriate changes to the practice or your systems.

The steps of a significant event audit are shown in Box 2.4.

Box 2.4:
Steps of a significant event audit

- *Step 1*: Describe who was involved, what time of day, what the task/activity was, the context and any other relevant information.
- *Step 2*: Reflect on the effects of the event on the participants and the professionals involved.
- *Step 3*: Discuss the reasons for the event or situation arising with other colleagues, review case notes or other records.
- *Step 4*: Decide how you or others might have behaved differently. Describe your options for how the procedures at work might be changed to minimise or eliminate the chances of the event recurring.

- *Step* 5: Plan changes that are needed, how they will be implemented, who will be responsible for what and when, what further training or resources are required. Then carry out the changes.
- *Step* 6: Re-audit later to see whether changes to procedures or new knowledge and skills are having the desired effects. Give feedback to the practice team.

An assessment by an external body

This is a traditional way of showing that you are competent by taking and passing an examination. It is a good way of testing recalled knowledge in a written or oral examination, or establishing how you behave in a clinical situation on the day of a practical examination, but not much good for measuring anything else. A summative examination (i.e. done at the end of a course of study) gives a measure of your learning up to that date.

You might undertake an objective test of your knowledge and skills. Examples are a computer-based test in the form of multiple choice questions and patient management problems as in the RCGP's phased evaluation programme (PEP) CD-ROMs (email pep@rcgp-scotland.org.uk) or the Apollo programme available from BMJ Publishing.[12] Various other organisations give multiple choice questionnaires that you can complete on paper and record in your portfolio.[13,14]

The RCGP's series of quality awards provide external assessment – Membership by Assessment of Performance, Fellowship by Assessment, Quality Team Development, etc. Trained assessors will give feedback to individual doctors or practice teams about their performance compared with set standards and their peers.

Elicit the views of patients

Part of meeting the criteria for relationships with patients in *Good Medical Practice*[5] might be to assess patients' satisfaction with:

- you
- your practice
- the local hospital's way of working
- other services available in your locality.

Avoid surveys where questions are relatively superficial or biased. A more specific enquiry should uncover particular elements of patients' dissatisfaction, which will be more useful if you are trying to identify your learning needs. Use a well-validated patient questionnaire, instead of risking producing your own version with ambiguities and flaws, such as the General Practice Assessment Questionnaire (GPAQ)[15] or the Doctors' Interpersonal Skills Questionnaire (DISQ).[16] Many doctors and practice teams have used these patient survey methods, providing a bank of data against which to compare your performance.

Other sources of feedback from patients might be obtained through suggestion boxes for patients to contribute comments, or the practice team recording all patients' suggestions and complaints, however trivial, looking for patterns in the comments received.

There will be learning to be had from every complaint – even if the complaint does not have any substance, there should be something to learn about the shortfall in communication between you and the complainant.

The evolution of the 'expert patient programme' should mean that there is a pool of well informed patients with chronic conditions who can contribute their insights into what you (or the service) need to learn from a patient's perspective.[17]

Strengths, weaknesses (or challenges), opportunities and threats (SWOT or SCOT) analysis

You can undertake a SWOT (or SCOT) analysis of your own performance or that of your practice team or practice organisation, working it out on your own, or with a workmate or mentor, or with a group of colleagues. Brainstorm the strengths, weaknesses (or challenges), opportunities and threats of your role or circumstances.

Strengths and weaknesses (or challenges) of your roles might relate to your clinical knowledge or skills, experience, expertise, decision making, communication skills, interprofessional relationships, political skills, timekeeping, organisational skills, teaching skills, or research skills. Strengths and weaknesses (or challenges) of the practice organisation might relate to most of these aspects as well as the way resources are allocated, overall efficiency and the degree to which the practice is patient centred.

Opportunities might relate to your unexploited experience or potential strengths, expected changes in the NHS, or resources for which you might bid. For example, you might train for and set up a special interest post.

Threats will include factors and circumstances that prevent you from achieving your aims for personal, professional and practice development or service improvements. They might be to do with your health, turnover in the practice team, or time-limited investment by the PCO.

List the important factors in your SWOT (or SCOT) analysis in order of priority through discussion with colleagues and independent people from outside your practice. Draw up goals and a timed action plan for you or the practice team to follow.

Informal conversations – in the corridor, over coffee

You learn such a lot when chatting with colleagues at coffee time or over a meal and can become aware of your learning or service development needs at these times. This is when you realise that other people are doing things differently from you, and if they seem to be doing it better and achieving more, you can challenge yourself to decide if this matter could be one of your blind spots. Note down your thoughts before you forget them so that you can reflect on them later.

Online discussion groups may provide another source of informal exchanges with colleagues. If you find this difficult to start with, you might 'lurk', viewing the comments and views of other people until you feel confident enough to contribute. Record any observations that you find useful and reflect on how they might inform your own practice.

Observe your work environment and role

Observation could be informal and opportunistic, or more systematic working through a structured checklist. One method of self-assessment might be to audiotape yourself at work dealing with patients (after obtaining patients' informed consent). Listen to the tape afterwards to appraise your communication and consultation skills – on your own or with a friend or colleague. If you have access to video equipment, you might use this instead.

Look at the equipment in your practice or your emergency bag. Do you know how to operate it properly? Assess yourself undertaking practical procedures or ask someone to watch you operate the equipment or undertaking the practical procedure and give you feedback about your performance.

Analyse the various roles and responsibilities of your current posts. Compare your level of expertise against national standards such as in the Knowledge and Skills Framework for England from the Department of Health or a job evaluation framework as part of the Agenda for Change initiative.[18,19] Determine if you can meet the requirements, or, if not, what deficiencies need to be made good.

You might combine one of the methods of identifying your learning needs already described such as an audit or SWOT analysis and apply it to 'observing your work environment or role', describing your relationship with other members of the multidisciplinary team for example, or reviewing how their roles and responsibilities interface with yours.

Read and reflect

When reading articles in respected journals, reflect on what the key messages mean for you in your situation. Note down topics about which you know little but that are relevant to your work, and calculate if you have further learning needs not met by the article you are reading. If the article is relevant to your practice, record what changes you will make and how you will make the changes. Record how you will impart your new knowledge to others in your practice.

Educational review

You might find a buddy or work colleague, CPD tutor, or a clinical tutor or clinical supervisor with whom you can have an informal or formal discussion about your performance, job situation and learning needs. You might draw up a learning contract as a result with a timed plan of action.

Identify your service needs – how you can find out if there are gaps in services or how you deliver care

Now focus your attention on the needs of your practice or the PCO. The standards of service delivery should be those that allow you to practise as a competent clinician. You may be competent but be unable to perform or practise to a competent level if the resources available to you are inadequate, or other colleagues have insufficient knowledge or skills to support you. You cannot be expected to take responsibility for ensuring that resources you need to be able to practise in a competent manner are available. However, as a professional you should play a significant role in collecting evidence to make a case for the need for essential resources to your GP colleagues, the practice manager, staff at the trust or PCO or whoever is appropriate.

Some of the methods you might use are described below and include:

- involving patients and the public in giving you feedback about the quality and quantity of your services

- monitoring access and availability to care
- undertaking a force-field analysis
- assessing risk
- evaluating the standards of care or services you provide
- comparing the systems in your practice with those required by legislation
- considering your patient population's health needs
- reviewing teamwork
- assessing the quality of your services
- reflecting on whether you are providing cost-effective care and services.

Involve patients and the public in giving you feedback about the quality and quantity of your services

Patient and public involvement may occur at three levels:

1 for individual patients about their own care
2 for patients and the public about the range and quality of health services on offer
3 in planning and organising health service developments.

The phrase 'patient and public involvement' is used here to mean individual involvement as a user, patient or carer, or public involvement that includes the processes of consultation and participation.[20]

If a patient involvement or public consultation exercise is to be meaningful, it has to involve people who represent the section of the population that the exercise is about. You will have to set up systems to actively seek out and involve people from minority groups or those with sensory impairments such as blind and deaf people.

Before you start:

- define the purpose
- be realistic about the magnitude of the planned exercise
- select an appropriate method or several methods depending on the target population and your resources
- obtain the commitment of everyone who will be affected by the exercise
- frame the method in accordance with your perspective
- write the protocol.

You might hold focus groups, or set up a patient panel, or invite feedback and help from a patient participation group. You could interview patients selected either at random from the patient population or for their experience of a particular condition or circumstance.

Monitor access to and availability of healthcare

Access and availability

You could look at waiting times to see a health professional by using:

- computerised appointment lists or paper and pen to record the time of arrival, the time of the appointment, the time seen
- the next available appointments that can easily be monitored by computer, or more painfully by manual searches of the appointment books.

Compare the results at intervals (a spreadsheet is a good way to do this). Do you or your staff have learning needs in relation to the use of technology, or new ways of redesigning the service you offer?

Referrals to other agencies and hospitals

You might audit and re-audit the time taken from the date the patient is seen to:

- the referral being sent (do you need more secretarial time?)
- the date the patient is seen by the other agency (could the patient be seen elsewhere quicker or do you need to liaise with other agencies over referrals?)
- the date the patient's needs have been met by investigation, diagnosis, treatment, provision of aid or support, etc (can you influence how quickly these are completed?).

Identify any learning needs here. For instance, new methods of teamwork with a different mix of skills between doctors, nurses and non-clinically qualified assistants could provide extra services in the practice, or you, or a colleague, might retrain to become a GP with a special clinical interest.

Draw up a force-field analysis

This tool will help you to identify and focus down on the positive and negative forces in your work and to gain an overview of the weighting of these factors. Draw a horizontal or vertical line in the middle of a sheet of paper. Label one side 'positive' and the other side 'negative'. Draw bars to represent individual positive drivers that motivate you on one side of the line, and factors that are demotivating on the other negative side of the line. The thickness and length of the bars should represent the extent of the influence; that is, a short, narrow bar will indicate that the positive or negative factor has a minor influence and a long, wide bar a major effect. *See* Box 2.5 for an example.

Box 2.5:   Example of force-field analysis diagram. Satisfaction with current post as a health professional

Positive factors (driving forces)	Negative factors (restraining forces)
career aspirations	long hours of work
salary	demands from patients
autonomy	
satisfaction from caring	job insecurity
no uniform	oppressive hierarchy
opportunities for professional development	

Take an overview of the resulting force-field diagram and consider if you are content with things as they are, or can think of ways to boost the positive side and minimise the negative factors. You can do this part of the exercise on your own, with a peer or a small group in the practice, or with a mentor or someone from outside the practice. The exercise should help you to realise the extent to which a known influence in your life, or in the practice as a whole, is a positive or negative factor. Make a personal or organisational action plan to create the situations and opportunities to boost the positive factors in your life and minimise the bars on the negative side.

Assess risk

Risk assessment might entail evaluating the risks to the health or wellbeing or competence of yourself, staff and/or patients in your practice or workplace, and deciding on the action needed to minimise or eliminate those risks.[21]

- *A hazard*: something with the potential to cause harm.
- *A risk*: the likelihood of that potential to cause harm being realised.

There are five steps to risk assessment:

1 look for and list the hazards
2 decide who might be harmed and how
3 evaluate the risks arising from the hazards and decide whether existing precautions are adequate or more should be done
4 record the findings
5 review your assessment from time to time and revise it if necessary.

You do not want to spend a lot of time and effort identifying risks or making changes if they do not matter much. When you have identified a risk, consider:

• is the risk large?
• does it happen often?
• is it a significant risk?

Risks may be prevented, avoided, minimised or managed where they cannot be eliminated. You, your colleagues and your staff may need to learn how to do this.

Record significant events where someone has experienced an adverse event or had a near miss – as part of you identifying your service development needs on an ongoing basis. Most significant incidents do not have one cause. Usually there are faults in the system, which are compounded by someone or several people being careless, tired, overworked or ill-informed. Cultivate an atmosphere of openness and discussion without blame so that you can all learn from the significant event. If people think they will be blamed they will hide the incident and no one will be able to prevent it happening again. Look for *all* the causes and try to remedy as many as possible to prevent the situation from arising in the future.

Evaluate the standards of services or care you provide

Keep your evaluation as simple as possible. Avoid wasting resources on unnecessarily bureaucratic evaluation. Design the evaluation so that you:

• specify the event (such as a service) to be evaluated – define broad issues, set priorities against strategic goals, time and resources, seek agreement on the nature and scope of the task
• describe the expected impact of the programme or activity and who will be affected
• define the criteria of success – these might relate to structure, process or outcome
• identify the information required to demonstrate the achievements of the programme or activity. The record might include: observing behaviour; data from existing records; prospective recording by the subjects of the programme or by the recipients and staff of the activity

- determine the time frame for the evaluation
- specify who collects the data for all stages in the delivery of the programme or activity, and the respective deadlines
- review and refine the objectives of the programme or activity and check that they are appropriate for the outcomes and impact you expect.

What to evaluate?

You could:

- adopt any, or all, of the six aspects of the health service's performance assessment framework (*see* Box 2.6)
- agree milestones and goals at stages in your programme or adopt others such as those relating to the National Service Frameworks for coronary heart disease or mental health
- evaluate the extent to which you achieve the outcome(s) starting with an objective. Alternatively, you might evaluate how conducive is the context of the programme, or activity, to achieving the anticipated outcomes
- undertake regular audits of aspects of the structure, process and outcome of a service or project to see if you have achieved what you expected when you established the criteria and standards of the audit programme
- evaluate the various components of a new system or programme: the activities, personnel involved, provision of services, organisational structure, precise goals and interventions.

Box 2.6:   The six aspects of the NHS performance assessment framework

1   Health improvement
2   Fair access
3   Effective delivery
4   Efficiency
5   Patient/carer experience
6   Health outcomes

Computer search

The extent to which you can evaluate your practice will depend on the quality of your records and extent to which you use the capacity of your practice computer. Compare the results of a computerised search for all those using one type of treatment with another. Make appropriate changes to your systems depending on what the computer search reveals. Put your plan into action and monitor with repeat searches at regular intervals.

Look at your learning or service development needs by analysing data from practice records to:

- look at trends and patterns of illness
- devise and use clinical guidelines and decision support systems as part of evidence-based practice
- audit what you are doing
- provide the information on which to base decisions on commissioning and management
- support epidemiology, research and teaching activities.

Compare the systems in your practice with those required by legislation

Legislation changes quite frequently. As an employer, a GP needs to keep abreast of the legislation or ensure that the practice manager does so. You could start by comparing the systems in your practice with those required by the Disability Discrimination Act (1995) and health and safety legislation.

Consider your patient population's health needs

Create a detailed profile of your practice population. Ask your PCO or public health lead for information about your practice population and comparative information about the general population living in the district – morbidity and mortality statistics, referral patterns, age/sex mix, ethnicity, and population trends.

Include information about the wider determinants of health such as housing, numbers of the population in, and types of, employment, geographical location, the environment, crime and safety, educational attainment and socioeconomic data. Make a note of any particular health problems such as higher than average teenage pregnancy rates or drug misuse. Focus on the current state of health inequalities within your practice population or between your practice population and the district as a whole. It may be that circumstances change, which in turn alters the proportion of minority groups in your practice population – such as if a continuing care home opens up in your practice area, or there is an influx of homeless people or asylum seekers into your locality.

Review teamwork

You can measure how effective the team is[22] – evaluate whether the team has:

- clear goals and objectives

- accountability and authority
- individual roles for members
- shared tasks
- regular internal formal and informal communication
- full participation by members
- confrontation of conflict
- feedback to individuals
- feedback about team performance
- outside recognition
- two-way external communication
- team rewards.

Assess the quality of your services

Quality may be subdivided into eight components: equity, access, acceptability and responsiveness, appropriateness, communication, continuity, effectiveness and efficiency.[23]

You might use the matrix in Box 2.7 as a way of ordering your approach to auditing a particular topic with the eight aspects of quality on the vertical axis and structure, process and outcome on the horizontal axis.[24] In this way you can generate up to 24 aspects of a particular topic. You might then focus on several aspects to look at the quality of patient care or services from various angles.

Box 2.7: Matrix for assessing the quality of a clinical service

You might look at the structure, process or outcome of communicating test results to patients for example.

	Structure	Process	Outcome
Equity			
Access			
Acceptability and responsiveness			
Appropriateness			
Communication	Hospital report	Feedback	Action taken
Continuity			
Effectiveness			
Efficiency			

Look for service development needs reflecting why patients receive a poor quality of service such as:

- inadequately trained staff or staff with poor levels of competence
- lack of confidentiality
- staff not being trained in the management of emergency situations
- doctors or nurses not being contactable in an emergency or being ineffective
- treatment being unavailable due to poor management of resources or services
- poor management of the arrangements for home visiting
- insufficient numbers of available staff for the workload
- qualifications of locums or deputising staff being unknown or inadequate for the posts they are filling
- arrangements for transfer of information from one team member to another being inadequate
- team members not acting on information received.

Many of these items will need action as a team, but for some of them, it may be your responsibility to ensure that adequate standards are met.

Reflect on whether you are providing cost-effective care and services

Cost-effectiveness is not synonymous with 'cheap'. A cost-effective intervention is one which gives a better or equivalent benefit from the intervention in question for lower or equivalent cost, or where the relative improvement in outcome is higher than the relative difference in cost. In other words being cost-effective means having the best outcomes for the least input. Using the term 'cost-effective' implies that you have considered potential alternatives.

An intervention must first be considered *clinically* effective to warrant investigation into its potential to be *cost*-effective. Evidence-based practice must incorporate clinical judgement. You have to interpret the evidence when it comes to applying it to individual patients, whether it is evidence about clinical effectiveness or cost-effectiveness. A new or alternative treatment or intervention should be compared directly with the previous best treatment or intervention.

An economic evaluation is a comparative analysis of two or more alternatives in terms of their costs and consequences. There are four different types as shown in Box 2.8.

Box 2.8:   The four types of economic evaluation

1   *Cost-effectiveness analysis* is used to compare the effectiveness of two interventions with the same treatment objectives.
2   *Cost minimisation* compares the costs of alternative treatments that have identical health outcomes.
3   *Cost–utility analysis* enables the effects of alternative interventions to be measured against a combination of life expectancy and quality of life; common outcome measures are quality adjusted life years (QALYs) or health-related quality of life (hrqol).
4   *Cost–benefit analysis* is a technique designed to determine the feasibility of a project, plan, management or treatment by quantifying its costs and benefits. It is often difficult to determine these accurately in relation to health.

While health valuation is unavoidable, it cannot be objective. You will probably have learning needs around what subjective method is best to use.[25]

Efficiency is sometimes confused with effectiveness. Being efficient means obtaining the most quality from the least expenditure, or the required level of quality for the least expenditure. To measure efficiency you need to make a judgement about the level of quality of the 'purchase' and be able to relate it to 'price'. 'Price' alone does not measure efficiency. Quality is the indicator used in combination with price to assess if something is more efficient. So, cost-effectiveness is a measure of efficiency and suggests that costs have been related to effectiveness.

Consider whether you have service development needs. Discuss whether:

• the current skill mix in your team is appropriate
• more cost-effective alternative types of delivery of care are available
• sufficient staff training exists for those taking on new roles and responsibilities.

Set priorities: how you match what's needed with what's possible

You and your colleagues will have been able to make a wish list after following the previous Stages 3A and 3B undertaking a variety of needs assessments. Group and summarise your learning and service development needs from the exercises you have carried out. Grade them according to the priority you set. You may put one at a higher priority because it fits in with learning needs established from another section, or put another lower because it does not fit in with other activities that you will put into your learning plan for the next

12 months. If you have identified a learning need by several different methods of assessment, then it will have a higher priority than something only identified once in your PDP. Collect information from all the team, the patients, users and carers to feed back before you make a decision on how to progress. Remember to consider external influences such as the National Service Frameworks, NICE guidance, governmental priorities, priorities of your PCO, the content of the Local Delivery Plan, etc.

Select those topics that are tied into organisational priorities, have clear aims and objectives and are achievable within your time and resource constraints. When ranking topics for learning or action in order of priority consider whether:

- your aims and objectives are clearly defined
- the topic is important:
  - for the population served (e.g. the size of the problem and/or its severity)
  - in relation to your skills, knowledge or attitudes
- it is feasible
- it is affordable
- learning about it will make enough difference
- learning fits in with other priorities.

You will still have more ideas than can possibly be implemented. Remember the highest priority – the health service is for patients that use it or who will do so in the future.

References

1   Medical Professionalism Project (2002) Medical professionalism in the new millennium: a physicians' charter. *Lancet.* **359:** 520–2.

2   www.gpwsi.org/subindex.shtml

3   Eraut M and du Boulay B (2000) *Developing the Attributes of Medical Professional Judgement and Competence.* University of Sussex, Sussex. Reproduced at www.cogs.susx.ac.uk/users/bend/doh/reporthtml.html

4   Fraser SW and Greenhalgh T (2001) Coping with complexity: educating for capability. *British Medical Journal.* **323:** 799–802.

5   General Medical Practice (2001) *Good Medical Practice.* General Medical Council, London.

6   Pendleton D, Schofield T, Tate P and Havelock P (2003) *The New Consultation, Developing Doctor–Patient Communication.* Oxford University Press, Oxford.

7   King J (2002) Career focus: 360° appraisal. *British Medical Journal.* **324:** S195.

8   Royal College of General Practitioners/General Practitioners Committee (2002) *Good Medical Practice for General Practitioners.* Royal College of General Practitioners, London.

9   National Institute for Clinical Excellence (NICE) www.nice.org.uk

10 Scottish Intercollegiate Guidelines Network (SIGN) www.sign.ac.uk

11 Irvine D and Irvine S (eds) (1991) *Making Sense of Audit.* Radcliffe Medical Press, Oxford.

12 Toon P, Greenhalgh T, Rigby M *et al.* (2002) *The Human Face of Medicine.* Two CD Roms in the APOLLO (Advancing Professional Practice through Online Learning Opportunities) series. BMJ Publishing Group, London. Free sample available at www.apollobmj.com

13 *Guidelines in Practice* www.eguidelines.co.uk

14 www.doctors.net.uk

15 www.npcrdc.man.ac.uk

16 www.ex.ac.uk/cfep

17 Department of Health (2003) *EPP Update newsletter.* Department of Health, London. See Expert Patient Programme on www.ohn.gov.uk/ohn/people/expert.htm

18 Department of Health (2004) *The NHS Knowledge and Skills Framework (NHS KSF) and Development Review Guidance – working draft.* Version 7. Department of Health, London.

19 Department of Health (2003) *Job Evaluation Handbook.* Version 1. Department of Health, London.

20 Chambers R, Drinkwater C and Boath E (2003) *Involving Patients and the Public: how to do it better* (2e). Radcliffe Medical Press, Oxford.

21 Mohanna K and Chambers R (2000) *Risk Matters in Healthcare.* Radcliffe Medical Press, Oxford.

22 Hart E and Fletcher J (1999) Learning how to change: a selective analysis of literature and experience of how teams learn and organisations change. *Journal of Interprofessional Care.* **13(1):** 53–63.

23 Maxwell RJ (1984) Quality assessment in health. *British Medical Journal.* **288:** 1470–2.

24 Firth-Cozens J (1993) *Audit in Mental Health Services.* LEA, Hove.

25 McCulloch D (2003) *Valuing Health in Practice.* Ashgate Publishing Ltd, Aldershot.

3

Demonstrating common components of good quality healthcare

In looking at the quality of care you provide and demonstrating your standards of service delivery and outcomes of learning, you should find that obtaining informed consent from patients for their treatment, maintaining confidentiality and handling complaints are part of the fabric of good quality care. We have considered them separately in this chapter, but each may be individualised to any of the seven clinical areas of Chapters 4 to 10.

We have set out the chapter with key information about consent followed by some example cycles of the stages of evidence (*see* Figure 1.1 on page 6). The two other sections on confidentiality and complaints follow, laid out in similar ways. Read through the cycles of evidence to become familiar with the approach to gathering and documenting evidence of your learning, competence, performance or standards of service delivery. Then either adopt one of the examples or adapt it to your own circumstances. Alternatively, read on to one or more of the clinical chapters and look at these three components in a clinical context such as in relation to asthma and chronic obstructive pulmonary disease in Chapters 4 and 5.

Consent

Key points

Information given to a health professional remains the property of the patient. In most circumstances, consent is assumed for the necessary sharing of information with other professionals involved with the care of the patient for that episode of care. Usually consent is also assumed for essential sharing of information for continuing care. Beyond this, informed consent must be obtained. Patients attend for healthcare in the belief that the personal information that they supply, or which is found out about them during investigation or treatment, will be confidential.

Exceptions to the above are:[1]

- if the patient consents
- if it is in the patient's own interest that information should be disclosed, but it is either impossible to seek the patient's consent or
- it is medically undesirable in the patient's own interest, to seek the patient's consent
- if the law requires (and does not merely permit) the health professional to disclose the information
- if the health professional has an overriding duty to society to disclose the information
- if the health professional agrees with a governmental agency that disclosure is necessary to safeguard national security
- if the disclosure is necessary to prevent a serious risk to public health
- in certain circumstances, for the purposes of medical research.

Health professionals must be able to justify their decision to disclose information without consent. If they are in any doubt, they should consult their professional bodies and colleagues.

Consent is only valid if the patient fully understands the nature and consequences of disclosure – they must be able to give their consent, receive enough information to enable them to make a decision and be acting under their own free will and not persuaded by the strong influence of another person. If consent is given, the health worker is responsible for limiting the disclosure to that information for which informed consent has been obtained. The development of modern information technology and the increasing amount of multidisciplinary teamwork in patient care make confidentiality difficult to uphold.

You may need to give information about a patient to a relative or carer. Normally the consent of the patient should be obtained. Sometimes, the clinical condition of the patient may prevent informed consent being obtained (e.g. they are unconscious or have a severe illness). It is important to recognise that relatives or carers do not have any right to information about the patient. Disclosure without consent may be justified when third parties are exposed to a risk so serious that it outweighs the patient's privacy. An example would be if a patient declines to allow you to disclose information about their health and continues to drive against medical advice when unfit to do so.

Local research ethics committees and the research governance framework ensure best practice in the giving of informed consent by patients in research studies.

As health professionals, we often assume implied consent. The general public and patients are generally ignorant of the extent to which information about them is passed around the NHS. When teaching at both undergraduate and postgraduate levels, in examinations and assessments and in research, we may incorrectly assume patients imply their consent. Consent is also implied for health service accounting, central monitoring of referrals, in disease registers, for audit and in facilitating joint working between team members. The NHS is still engaged in a debate about what data can legitimately be shared without patients' explicit consent. Although written consent is usually obtained for supplying information to insurance companies or for legal reports, patients are often unaware of the type of information being supplied and have not given 'informed consent'. Guidelines published jointly by the British Medical Association (BMA) and the Association of British Insurers clarify that doctors are not required to release all aspects of a patient's medical history but need only submit (with the patient's consent) information that is relevant.[2]

The GMC's booklet *Seeking Patients' Consent: the ethical considerations* explores issues of consent in more depth and advises that:

> the amount of information you give each patient will vary according to factors such as the nature of the condition, the complexity of the treatment, the risks associated with the treatment or procedure and the patient's own wishes . . . you should be careful about relying on a patient's apparent compliance with a procedure as a form of consent.[3]

Collecting data to demonstrate your learning, competence, performance and standards of service delivery: consent

Example cycle of evidence 3.1

- Focus: informed consent
- Other relevant focus: research

Stages of the evidence cycle

Stage 1
Select targets

Stage 2
Set standards

Stage 5
Document it all

Stage 3A/B
Identify needs

Stage 4
Learning/action plan

Case study 3.1

You agree as a practice to undertake a survey to find out if patients are satisfied with your service. The practice manager will organise it, but you are nominated to lead the work. You decide to focus on teenagers as a group as the adolescent drop-in clinic you set up two years ago with the school health service is not being used as much as it once was. You want to be proactive about helping teenagers resist smoking and drugs, encourage healthy eating and exercise, protect their mental health and encourage their management of chronic diseases such as asthma and diabetes, etc. You are not sure how to survey the teenagers. You think they are unlikely to answer questionnaires sent through the post and think you will interview teenagers about their satisfaction with the clinic. You intend to employ one of your own teenage children to interview some who have never come to the clinic, by selecting their names from your patient list as well as some teenagers who have attended. You're not sure if you are getting into research territory or if it is okay to claim you are auditing your services.

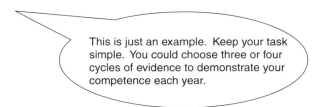

This is just an example. Keep your task simple. You could choose three or four cycles of evidence to demonstrate your competence each year.

Stage 1: Select your aspirations for good practice

The excellent GP:

- protects patients' rights and makes sure that they are not disadvantaged by taking part in research
- gives patients the information they need about their problem in a way they can understand as a basis for informed consent.

Stage 2: Set the standards for your outcomes

Outcomes might include:

- the way learning is applied
- a learnt skill
- a protocol
- a strategy that is implemented
- meeting recommended standards.

- The informed consent policy of the practice covers patients' participation in audit and research as well as consent to clinical treatment.
- You are able to describe the difference between what is audit of clinical management and service provision and what is research.

Stage 3A: Identify your learning needs

- Read through the frequently asked questions and answers on the Department of Health website relating to research governance.[4] Consider whether you are able to answer the questions before reading the answers.
- Describe an audit plan of an adolescent clinic that involves obtaining young people's views of standards of services by interviewing them. Submit the plan to the chair of the local research ethics committee to check that he/she agrees that the audit proposal does not fall within the definition of research and to approve the patient literature and the process inviting informed consent to take part.

- Self-assess your own knowledge about teenagers consenting to treatment or research, and identify any differences in your approach if they are under or over the age of 16 years.

Stage 3B: Identify your service needs

> Any of the needs assessment exercises in 3A may also reveal service needs.

- Draw up an information leaflet for young people about the audit of adolescent clinic services that you intend to carry out. Ask others to critique the leaflet – young people for its readability and clarity, a research colleague for the extent to which it conforms to best practice for informed consent. Use the information leaflet so that they can give informed consent to the interview to obtain their views and an audio recording of the interview.
- Ask a colleague to peer review the extent to which advice and information you give to teenagers during a consultation is accurate. The teenager would need to have given prior, written informed consent for the peer review (and audio recording if used).

Stage 4: Make and carry out a learning and action plan

- Obtain and read the documents about research governance from the Department of Health's website or from your PCO – as in section 3A first point.[4]
- Study the application form for the ethical approval of a research study.
- Understand the limits to obtaining patients' views as part of audit of clinical and service management by reading up on informed consent. Read the GMC's booklet: *Seeking Patients' Consent: the ethical considerations.*[3] Look at whether you are explaining the details of the diagnosis or prognosis, giving an explanation of likely benefits and side-effects, explaining whether a proposed treatment is experimental and whether a doctor in training will be involved.
- Ask for a short tutorial from your local clinical governance lead about good practice in obtaining patients' views through audit, research and patient involvement activities – including good practice in informed consent and any special considerations for teenagers aged under 16 years.

Stage 5: Document your learning, competence, performance and standards of service delivery

- Keep a comparison of your own practice with the answers to the frequently asked questions on the Department of Health website relating to research governance.[4]
- File a copy of the response letter from the chair of local research ethics committee about the audit proposal.
- Document that the subsequent revised audit plan shows that the work does not fall within the definition of research.
- Keep a copy of the revised teenage patients' informed consent leaflet, following the critique.
- Repeat the peer review by the same, or another, colleague of the extent to which advice and information you give to teenagers during consultations is accurate.

Case study 3.1 continued

The chair of the research ethics committee advises you that your plan should be classed as research rather than audit as it involves contact with patients outside their usual NHS care. He explains about the risks of using untrained interviewers such as your own children, and the need to fully inform those teenagers you are inviting to be interviewed about the survey and that their refusal will not prejudice their medical care. He advises you to send an application form for formal approval to the ethics committee and to contact the research lead in your PCO in line with the research governance framework if you wish to continue to develop a research project. You revise your plans as the scale of the work required is becoming out of all proportion.

Confidentiality

Key points

You should have appropriate confidentiality safeguards in place in the practice to prevent inadvertent disclosure of personal and sensitive information about patients. Tell people, especially the young, about their right to confidential medical treatment and reinforce your conversation with posters and leaflets. People with non-prescription drug-related problems who seek help from substance abuse clinics, or those with sexually transmitted infections who attend genitourinary medicine clinics, often do not want their GP to be told because they do not believe that the information will be kept confidential. Fears about confidentiality are the commonest reason young people give for not attending their general practitioner for contraceptive treatment.[5]

Young people under the age of 16 years have the same rights to confidentiality as other patients. The younger the person, the greater care is needed to assess the level of understanding to ensure that he or she understands the consequences of any proposed action. If a young person fulfils the conditions of the Fraser Guidelines (England and Wales) he or she is regarded as being competent to make his or her own decisions.[6] In Scotland, the Age of Legal Capacity (Scotland) Act 1991 gives similar powers of consent to those under 16 years of age. In Northern Ireland separate legislation applies.

Occasionally you may feel that you have a moral obligation to divulge confidential information. Whenever possible you should seek to persuade the patient to give consent to the disclosure. Seek advice from your professional organisations in circumstances where others are at danger (e.g. risk of harm, or rape or sexual abuse), or where a serious crime has been committed. Health professionals should satisfy themselves that sufficient authority has been obtained (e.g. a certificate from the Attorney General or Lord Advocate) and consult professional organisations before disclosing information without a patient's consent.

The Caldicott Committee Report described principles of good practice to safeguard confidentiality when information is being used for non-clinical purposes:[7]

- justify the purpose
- do not use patient-identifiable information unless it is absolutely necessary
- use the minimum necessary patient-identifiable information
- access to patient-identifiable information should be on a strict need-to-know basis
- everyone with access to patient-identifiable information should be aware of his or her responsibilities.

Interpreters should be used wherever possible to avoid the use of friends or relatives. They should be trained in the requirements of confidentiality.

Patients are entitled to access data held about them. Exceptions to this right are:

- the patient failed to make the request in accordance with the Data Protection Act 1998
- if acceding to the request would result in disclosure of information about somebody else without their consent
- when giving medical information may cause serious harm to the mental or physical health of the patient (a rare occurrence).

You need to incorporate systems for ensuring that paper and computer security are maintained. Systems for monitoring and upgrading security systems should be in place and you should check regularly that confidentiality is not being breached if changes are made.

Collecting data to demonstrate your learning, competence, performance and standards of service delivery: confidentiality

Example cycle of evidence 3.2

- Focus: confidentiality
- Other relevant focus: teaching and training

Stages of the evidence cycle

Stage 1
Select targets

Stage 2
Set standards

Stage 5
Document it all

Stage 3A/B
Identify needs

Stage 4
Learning/action plan

Case study 3.2

It is the first time you have had medical students placed with you and you want to teach two of them about the importance of making sure that student visitors understand the practice code on confidentiality while they are on their placement with you.

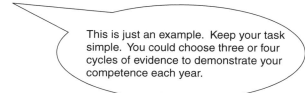

This is just an example. Keep your task simple. You could choose three or four cycles of evidence to demonstrate your competence each year.

Stage 1: Select your aspirations for good practice

The excellent GP:

- maintains the confidentiality of patient-specific information
- ensures that patients are not put at risk when seeing students or doctors in training.

Stage 2: Set the standards for your outcomes

Outcomes might include:

- the way learning is applied
- a learnt skill
- a protocol
- a strategy that is implemented
- meeting recommended standards.

- Ensure that all members of the practice team, including you, new members of staff and students or doctors in training, are familiar with guidelines for confidentiality in relation to patients receiving healthcare.

Stage 3A: Identify your learning needs

- Assess your knowledge about the limits of confidentiality, e.g. for providing under-16 year olds with contraception or divulging information about the health of patients with dementia to relatives or carers.
- Ask an expert tutor's opinion about the particular method of teaching you plan to use for an in-house training session. The session will be on maintaining confidentiality for teenagers of different ages and people with varying severity of mental health problems. It should convey the main messages and lead to changes where necessary.

Stage 3B: Identify your service needs

> Any of the needs assessment exercises in 3A may also reveal service needs.

- Compare the practice protocol for confidentiality with the guidelines in the *Confidentiality and Young People* toolkit.[5]
- Review your current or the intended induction programme for new members of staff, students on placement and doctors in training, to assess the extent to which knowledge of confidentiality features and is addressed.
- Organise a test of several different examples of patient episodes for members of the practice team, where confidentiality is complex and students or staff may be uncertain about the correct approach, based on the frequently asked questions on confidentiality published by the GMC.[8,9]

Stage 4: Make and carry out a learning and action plan

- Find out from the local educational tutor how to undertake learning needs assessments of others from different disciplines with different levels of responsibilities in respect of confidentiality.
- Prepare for and run an interactive teaching session on confidentiality for patients of all age groups and conditions. You might invite the whole practice team, including students, family planning or school nurses, local pharmacists, GP registrars, etc. You could use the *Confidentiality and Young People* toolkit and the answers to the GMC's frequently asked questions, for promoting discussion with the practice team at the session.[5,8,9]

Stage 5: Document your learning, competence, performance and standards of service delivery

- Keep the answers of the quiz completed by those attending the teaching session before and after their training about confidentiality.
- Keep an incident record kept by the practice team of any reported or perceived breaches of confidentiality by anyone working in, or associated with, the practice.
- Include examples of personal learning plans based on learning needs assessments for new staff or doctors in training by the end of their induction period.
- Include the revised practice protocol in line with the *Confidentiality and Young People* toolkit and GMC guidance on confidentiality.[5,8,9]

Case study 3.2 continued

Other staff colleagues join your teaching session with the students using the video from the *Confidentiality and Young People* toolkit.[5] All get full marks in the quiz after watching the video. The frequently asked questions published by the GMC really enhance their understanding about how confidentiality issues are managed in practice.[8,9]

Learning from complaints

Key points

There is learning to be had from every complaint. The GMC received a record 5539 complaints in 2002, 4% more than in 2001; of these, 72 resulted in a doctor being banned or suspended.[10] Even if the complaint is trivial or undeserved, it implies a lack of communication. Table 3.1 describes the nature of claims against GPs reported in a study of 1000 consecutive clinical cases. There are a myriad of associated reasons for the claims. Many of the clinical events will reveal failings in the practice systems and processes and in the practice of the GP – such as communication, diagnostic skills, etc.

Table 3.1:   Nature of 1000 claims against GPs handled by the Medical Protection Society[11]

Claim by patient	Number of claims
Problems of diagnosis (delayed or missed)	631
Prescribing errors	193
Malignant neoplasms (some of the problems of diagnosis)	140
Cancer of the breast (lumpiness often falsely diagnosed as benign)	20
Cancer of the cervix (often abnormalities are filed away and not acted upon)	14
Cancer of the digestive organs (cancer of colon most frequent with misdiagnosed symptoms)	21
Diabetes (8 deaths) primary failure to diagnose (19 delays in diagnosis; 9 delays in referral of patient resulting in amputation)	40
Myocardial infarction 27 deaths (8 undiagnosed, 7 diagnosed as dyspepsia; 3 diagnosed as congestive cardiac failure; 3 as muscular origin; 2 as chest infection)	34
Prescribing	
Steroids (e.g. osteoporotic collapse)	40
Antibiotic allergy	8
Phenothiazines (extrapyramidal symptoms)	10
Hormone replacement therapy	9
Oral contraception	9
Warfarin (interactions e.g. resulting in cerebral haemorrhage)	5

Collecting data to demonstrate your learning, competence, performance and standards of service delivery: complaints

Example cycle of evidence 3.3

- Focus: complaints
- Other relevant focus: working with colleagues

Stages of the evidence cycle

Stage 1
Select targets

Stage 2
Set standards

Stage 5
Document it all

Stage 3A/B
Identify needs

Stage 4
Learning/action plan

Case study 3.3

Your practice has received a patient complaint about a GP locum failing to diagnose a patient's thyroid cancer on the first occasion they consulted. This has prompted you all as a practice team to review the way that your complaints system functions.

This is just an example. Keep your task simple. You could choose three or four cycles of evidence to demonstrate your competence each year.

Stage 1: Select your aspirations for good practice

The excellent GP:

- apologises appropriately when things go wrong, and has an adequate complaints procedure in place.

Stage 2: Set the standards for your outcomes

> Outcomes might include:
>
> - the way learning is applied
> - a learnt skill
> - a protocol
> - a strategy that is implemented
> - meeting recommended standards.

- Understand and establish effective processes for preventing and managing complaints from patients in the practice.

Stage 3A: Identify your learning needs

- Examine as a significant event one or more complaints, e.g. where the practice has not advised a patient correctly about the complaints process.
- Compare the actual care of a patient against an acceptable standard of care for a range of clinical conditions as an ongoing review for a clinical area that has been the subject of a complaint (e.g. thyroid cancer in the case study). You could use peer review by asking respected colleagues, or compare your practice against a published standard such as a guideline by a responsible body of professional opinion.

Stage 3B: Identify your service needs

> Any of the needs assessment exercises in 3A may also reveal service needs.

- Audit patient complaints in the preceding 12 months: the number, the outcomes and how the complaint system is advertised, etc.
- Audit the extent to which doctors and nurses are following practice agreed protocols. Be proactive about preventing or minimising the likelihood of the source of the complaint recurring.

- Audit vulnerable areas. Look back at the analysis of complaints to identify useful areas for focusing learning, e.g. a review of the prescribing of steroids.
- Review the way that the qualifications of locums are checked and that they are made aware of the practice protocols.

Stage 4: Make and carry out a learning and action plan

- Ask your PCO to look at the practice complaints system and feed back how it can be improved (if at all).
- Arrange a tutorial between the practice manager and others in the team about preventing and managing complaints, or use one of the risk management packages produced by medical defence organisations.[12,13]
- Read up on how to undertake significant event analysis including how to share the information with the practice team and respond as a practice team.

Stage 5: Document your learning, competence, performance and standards of service delivery

- Include evidence of clinical competence to guard against a complaint.
- Include the protocol of the patient complaint process against which consecutive complaints can be audited in another 12 months' time.
- Record the guidance about physical examinations, including that the reason for any examination should be communicated clearly, that a chaperone should be offered for any internal or breast examination, and the comfort and privacy of the patient should always be kept in mind to avoid potential complaints.
- Record that a file containing practice protocols is available for easy reference on the desktop of the computer.

Case study 3.3 continued

You are invited by your PCO to take a lead in advising GPs in other practices about the handling of complaints because they were impressed by the way your complaint system was applied when you invited them to visit your practice and advise about the handling of complaints.

References

1   Chambers R and Wakley G (2000) *Making Clinical Governance Work for You.* Radcliffe Medical Press, Oxford.

2   British Medical Association and Association of British Insurers (2002) *Medical Information and Insurance.* British Medical Association, London. See www.bma. org.uk/ap.nsf/Content/MedicalInfoInsurance

3   General Medical Council (2002) *Seeking Patients' Consent: the ethical considerations.* General Medical Council, London.

4   www.dh.gov.uk/PolicyAnd Guidance/ResearchAnd Development/fs/en

5   Royal College of General Practitioners and Brook (2000) *Confidentiality and Young People. A toolkit for general practice, primary care groups and trusts.* Royal College of General Practitioners, London.

6   The Fraser Guidelines (1985) House of Lords Judgement, London.

7   Department of Health (1997) Report of the review of patient-identifiable information. In: *The Caldicott Committee Report.* Department of Health, London.

8   General Medical Council (2004) *Confidentiality: protecting and providing information.* General Medical Council, London.

9   General Medical Council (2004) *Frequently Asked Questions. Confidentiality: protecting and providing information.* General Medical Council, London. See www.gmc-uk.org for updated questions and answers.

10 General Medical Council (2003) *Fitness to Practise Statistics for 2002.* General Medical Council, London.

11 Panting G (2003) *Nature of 1000 Claims against GPs.* Medical Protection Society, London (presentation at primary care conference, Birmingham).

12 MPS Risk Consulting, Granary Wharf House, Leeds LS11 5PY or www.mps-riskconsulting.com

13 MDU Services Ltd, 230 Blackfriars Road, London SE1 8PJ or www.the-mdu.com

4

Asthma

This chapter discusses the management of asthma in adults. It is beyond the scope of this chapter to give a complete description of the management of all aspects of asthma. This task is far better served by reference to publications such as the SIGN and the British Thoracic Society guideline on the management of asthma.[1]

Case study 4.1

Ms Stub, a 23-year-old student, presents in surgery with a several month history of a troublesome cough. The cough is intermittent, but has been more noticeable over the past few days. It tends to be worse at night and is often accompanied by a wheeze and a slight sensation of not being able to get her breath. She smokes 15 cigarettes a day. She tells you that she suffered from eczema as a child. Her father suffered from hay fever and an elder brother has asthma. She wonders if her symptoms could indicate that she has asthma too.

What issues you should cover

The symptoms of asthma are:

* wheeze
* shortness of breath
* chest tightness
* cough.

These will tend to be variable, intermittent, worse at night and provoked by triggers including exercise.[1] Ms Stub presents three of these four symptoms. Her symptoms are variable and tend to be worse at night. She also gives both a family history and personal history of atopy. The presence of these symptoms and factors suggest, but do not conclusively prove, a diagnosis of asthma.

Case study 4.1 continued

You examine Ms Stub. She has a slightly red throat and generalised enlarged cervical glands. Her temperature is 37.5°C. Her pulse is 86/min in sinus rhythm, her blood pressure (BP) is 136/84 mmHg, auscultation of her chest is clear. At 1.67 m tall, her peak flow rate is 450 l/min with a predicted peak flow rate of 490 l/min.

Ms Stub's history as given is consistent with a diagnosis of asthma. Sometimes a mild respiratory tract infection will sufficiently worsen the asthma and bring the patient to the surgery. The respiratory tract infection and the history of smoking are both 'confounding' factors that may produce cough, chest tightness and shortness of breath.

Her peak expiratory flow rate (PEFR) is 92% of that predicted for a female of her age and height. This figure in isolation does not aid diagnosis, as diagnosis of adult asthma is based on demonstrating variance of the PEFR over time and throughout the day. You explain to Ms Stub that she has a mild viral infection. Antibiotics would (unfortunately) not speed recovery. You advise that she takes paracetamol and fluids.

You explain that, although asthma may account for her longer-term symptoms, you are not in a position to diagnose this as asthma – yet. You feel that the best way to confirm or exclude a diagnosis of asthma is for her to measure her peak flow over the next few days and then you will see her again with the results of this. You explain that she should check her peak flow twice daily and when she feels wheezy or short of breath. She should take three attempts at each measurement and record the best score of these as her peak flow. This should be recorded in her peak flow diary.

You demonstrate how to use the peak flow meter and ask Ms Stub to demonstrate to you how she will measure her peak flow, to ensure that she has acquired sufficient technique to accurately measure her PEFR. Then you prescribe a peak flow meter.

You also use the opportunity to discuss the importance of her stopping smoking. You offer to refer her for smoking cessation guidance and support but she declines.

Definitions used in respiratory function testing

You may come across a bewildering variety of expressions used to describe abnormalities of respiratory function. Some of the common ones are shown in Box 4.1.

Box 4.1: Common definitions used in describing respiratory function

- **Ventilation (*V*):** movement of air into and out of the respiratory passage ways
- **Tidal volume (V_T):** amount of air exhaled in a single normal breath (about 500 ml at rest)
- **Breathing frequency (*f*) or respiratory rate (RR):** the number of breaths per minute (about 12 at rest)
- **Minute ventilation ($\dot{V}$):** movement of air into and out of the lungs per minute (measured in l/min)
  for example: $\dot{V} = V_T \times f$ so at rest $\dot{V} = 500$ ml $\times 12 = 6000$ ml/min
- **Alveolar ventilation ($\dot{V}_A$):** volume of air that enters the alveoli and participates in gas exchange (respiratory zone)
- **Dead space:** area where no gas exchange takes place
- **Anatomical dead space (V_D):** volume of air in the conducting zone (about 150 ml/breath)
- **Physiological dead space:** areas of no gas exchange due to disease

Evaluation of pulmonary function through the measurement of vital capacity and peak flow:

- **Forced vital capacity (FVC):** maximal amount of air exhaled after a maximal inspiration (measured in litres)
- **Peak expiratory flow rate (PEFR):** maximal rate of air flow during a forced expiration (l/min)
- **Forced expiratory volume in 1 s (FEV_1):** amount of air expired in the first second of a maximal expiration
- **FEV_1/FVC:** ratio of volume of air expired in one second to the total volume of air maximally expired

---

Reversibility tests

The patient's condition should be stable (i.e. at least six weeks from an exacerbation) when performing diagnostic reversibility tests. Before a bronchodilator reversibility test, the patient must be asked to stop their short acting beta$_2$-agonist for 6 h, long-acting bronchodilator for 12 h and theophyllines for 24 h. Then:

- perform baseline spirometry
- give a bronchodilator (e.g. nebulised salbutamol 2.5 mg)
- after 15 min perform post-bronchodilator spirometry

- use a trial of oral steroids (30–40 mg daily for 2 weeks) for patients with obstructive lung disease who have an FEV_1 less than 60% of predicted.

Significant reversibility is defined as a rise in FEV_1 that is *both* greater than 200 ml *and* 15% of the pre-test value. Substantial reversibility (more than 500 ml) indicates asthma.

   See Chapter 5 on chronic obstructive pulmonary disease for more information about spirometry. You could also look at a useful paper illustrating the use of the symptoms and testing in the primary care diagnosis of cough.[2]

Exercise testing

Exercise testing is quite difficult to organise in primary care unless you are fortunate enough to have static exercise equipment in your practice. You could substitute stair climbing or corridor walking, but this is difficult to standardise.

Diagnosing asthma

The process for diagnosis of asthma is summarised in Box 4.2.

Box 4.2: Diagnosis of asthma

Asthma may be diagnosed in adults by the following criteria (taken from British guidelines on the management of asthma)[1]

- *Symptoms*: episodic/variable: cough, wheeze, shortness of breath, chest tightness
- *Signs*: wheeze, increased breathing frequency (but there are often no signs)
- *Additional information*:
    - personal or family history of atopy
    - symptoms worsen following use of aspirin, non-steroidal anti-inflammatory drugs (NSAIDs) or beta-blockers
    - recognised triggers: pollens, dust, animals, exercise, viral infection, chemical irritants
    - pattern and severity of symptoms and exacerbations
- *Objective measurements* (**one** of the following is diagnostic):
    - more than 20% diurnal variation on at least three days a week in two successive weeks in the peak flow diary

---

- FEV$_1$ is increased by at least 15% (and 200 ml) after taking a short-acting beta$_2$-agonist (e.g. salbutamol 400 µg by metered dose inhaler in a spacer or 2.5 mg via nebuliser)
- FEV$_1$ increased by at least 15% (and 200 ml) after a trial of steroid tablets (e.g. prednisolone 30 mg/day for 14 days)
- FEV$_1$ is decreased by at least 15% after six minutes of exercise.

Case study 4.1 continued

Two weeks later Ms Stub returns with her peak flow diary. Her peak flow readings show a variance between her highest and lowest daily measurements of at least 23% on four days during the first week and five days during the second week. You explain that, as this shows a greater than 20% diurnal variation on at least three days per week of two successive weeks, this is diagnostic of asthma.

Having told Ms Stub that she has asthma, there are now several tasks for you to perform. These are:

- patient education: theory
- treatment
- patient education: skills
- follow up
- health promotion
- patient empowerment.

Patient education: theory

Generally, people are more likely to follow an agreed plan if they understand the reasoning behind the plan. Ask Ms Stub to tell you what she already knows about asthma. As she has a brother with the condition she is likely to be somewhat familiar with the condition, but you may need to correct some misconceptions. It is important that her understanding and your approach coincide. Once a patient has a good mental 'model' of a disease, they can make informed choices regarding the management of their disease.

Treatment of asthma

Consider which drugs to recommend and which devices would be best to deliver these drugs. In this case, a salbutamol metered dose inhaler (MDI) to be used as required and a beclometasone 200 mg MDI to be used regularly twice daily will be appropriate.

Explain your recommendations for treatment to the patient. Discuss the role that each of these inhalers will play in the management of her asthma. Box 4.3 gives guidelines for the treatment of adult asthma.

Box 4.3:   Guidelines for the treatment of asthma in adults

The British Thoracic Society[3] and SIGN[4] have produced a stepwise summary of the (pharmacological) management of asthma in adults reproduced below.[1]

Treatment should be commenced at the step that seems most appropriate to the severity of the patient's asthma. The treatment may be stepped up or stepped down as dictated by the response and severity of the patient's asthma. The dose of inhaled steroid given refers to beclometasone diproprionate or equivalent.

Step 1: mild intermittent asthma

- Inhaled short-acting beta$_2$-agonist as required

Step 2: regular preventer therapy

- Add inhaled steroid 200–800 µg/day

Step 3: add-on therapy

- Add inhaled long-acting beta$_2$-agonist (LABA)
- Assess control of asthma:
  - good response to LABA: continue LABA
  - benefits from LABA but control still inadequate: continue LABA and increase inhaled steroid dose to 800 µg a day
  - no response to LABA: stop LABA and increase inhaled steroid to 800 µg/day. If control still inadequate, institute trial of other therapies e.g. leukotriene receptor antagonist, sustained release theophylline

Step 4: persistent poor control

- Consider trials of:
  - increasing inhaled steroid up to 2000 µg/day
  - addition of fourth drug e.g. leukotriene receptor antagonist, sustained release theophylline, or oral beta$_2$-agonist

> **Step 5: continuous or frequent use of oral steroids**
>
> - Use daily steroid dose in lowest dose providing adequate control
> - Maintain high-dose inhaled steroid at 2000 µg /day
> - Consider other treatments to minimise steroid use
> - Refer patient to specialist care

Patient education: skills

As Ms Stub has agreed to your recommendations, make sure that she learns the skills necessary to use the treatment in an optimal way. You may teach her yourself or ask an appropriately trained and experienced practice nurse to do so. Do not neglect this aspect as inadequate technique contributes to poor control of symptoms. Many people find the asthma website helpful in re-inforcing how to use their inhalers, using a spacer, what types are available (e.g. metered dose, breath-actuated or dry powder) and for tips such as not storing dry powder devices in the bathroom (as they clog up).[5]

Follow-up

This has two aspects: formalised follow-up at the practice, perhaps at the practice asthma clinic; and the monitoring that Ms Stub herself will be carrying out of her condition. This will include an appreciation of relevant symptoms, report on how frequently reliever treatment is used and peak flow rates during her daily life.

Health promotion

Certain lifestyle changes are beneficial in minimising asthma: these are smoking cessation and weight reduction. Both of these require the patient to be ready to change. All the practice team should give support and encouragement.

Patient empowerment

This means enabling the patient to feel in control of their illness and its management.

This should have been already partially achieved following the education given to the patient regarding their asthma. If Ms Stub feels able to take an active role in the monitoring of her condition, she will feel more in control. Then agree a patient-held asthma management plan together, so that Ms Stub knows what to do in response to differing peak flow rates and symptoms. She can utilise the data collected by her self-monitoring of symptoms, peak flow rates and response to treatment.

Lastly, put the patient in touch with asthma self-help groups, such as the National Asthma Campaign.[5]

Case study 4.1 continued

Ms Stub concurs with your management suggestions and quickly masters using her inhalers to best effect. She agrees to attend the nurse-run smoking cessation clinic at your practice. You both agree on an asthma management plan, which is personalised to Ms Stub's peak flow readings and treatment. She agrees to return for follow up at the practice's nurse-led asthma clinic in one month's time where the practice nurse covers the areas described below.

Asthma review in general practice-based asthma clinic

The practice nurse will build up a good working relationship with Ms Stub so that they can work together to minimise the effects the asthma has on her lifestyle.

Opinions vary as to the fine detail that should be covered in a standard asthma review. An example is as follows:

History

- What symptoms is the patient experiencing:
  - difficulty sleeping because of asthma symptoms?
  - any daytime symptoms (cough/wheeze/breathlessness/chest tightness)?
  - has asthma interfered with the patient's usual activity?
- What treatment(s) is the patient using?
  - how often is reliever inhaler required?
- Do any factors trigger asthma attacks?
- Smoking status.
- Date of the last asthma attack.
- Has the patient required hospitalisation?
- Has the patient required emergency steroids?

Examination

- Check the patient's peak flow.
- Examine the patient's peak flow diary.
- Check the patient's inhaler technique.

Patient education

- Discuss smoking if relevant (consider referral to smoking cessation clinic).
- Discuss the nature and avoidance of trigger factors.
- Reinforce good inhaler technique.
- Address other appropriate health promotion areas e.g. maintaining reasonable weight and taking regular exercise.

Review or modify treatment (the degree of responsibility taken by the nurse depends on her training and capabilities)

- Review treatment: step up or down as appropriate (*see* Boxes 4.3 and 4.4).
- If required, modify the inhaler device used and teach the patient the correct technique for the new inhaler device.
- Review the patient-held asthma management plan and modify if necessary (*see* British guidelines on the management of asthma[3,4] for example of a personal asthma diary and action plan – many pharmaceutical companies supply them).

Update patient and practice records accordingly. Ensure that the data collected in the practice's asthma clinic also allows ready audit of these areas in relation to the new GMS contract for GPs' quality and outcomes framework (*see* page 68).[6]

Box 4.4 describes the background to making decisions at an asthma review about increasing or decreasing a patient's treatment depending on their previous response and degree of control of asthma. The decision as to whether a patient's treatment should be stepped up or stepped down is based on how well controlled that patient's asthma is. The aim of 'perfect' control should be to some extent balanced against side-effects and difficulties of treatment and in maintaining a reasonable lifestyle. If a patient's control is suboptimal then stepping up treatment should be considered. When control (by the criteria at review in the asthma clinic) is very good, then stepping down treatment may be considered.

Box 4.4:   Stepping up and stepping down asthma treatment[1]

Control of asthma is assessed against the following criteria:

- minimal symptoms during day and night
- minimal need for reliever medication
- no exacerbations
- no limitation of physical activity
- actual versus expected lung function (in practical terms FEV_1 and/or PEFR more than 80% predicted or best).

When deciding which drug to step down first, and at what rate, consider the severity of the asthma, the side-effects of treatment, how effective each drug is, and the preferences of the patient.

   Patients should be on the lowest dose of inhaled steroids that controls their asthma. If feasible, reduce the inhaled steroid dose by about a quarter to a half but no quicker than every three months.

Case study 4.1 continued

On review at the asthma clinic, Ms Stub tells the nurse that she has rarely had any symptoms. She is using her beclometasone regularly. She has only required salbutamol on average twice weekly. She is also attending the nurse-led smoking cessation clinic. Her peak flow diary shows PEFR recorded as between 470 and 490 l/min. Peak flow on examination at the clinic is 480 l/min. Her inhaler technique is good. The nurse discusses her asthma management plan with her and Ms Stub demonstrates a clear understanding of it.

Management of acute asthma

Case study 4.2

During a relatively quiet July evening surgery, you are somewhat surprised to see Mr Dram. He is a 34-year-old unemployed man who rarely attends. He was last seen six months ago with alcohol dependency for which he was referred to a specialist but defaulted on his appointment. He smells of alcohol, but does not appear intoxicated. Looking at his notes, you see that he has had occasional prescriptions for a salbutamol inhaler, having been diagnosed with asthma some 15 years ago. Despite invitations to the practice's asthma clinic he has never attended for a review of his asthma.

He wants some antibiotics for his cough and a prescription for another salbutamol inhaler, 'perhaps a stronger one . . . this one . . . doesn't seem to . . . be working properly'. It is apparent from his interrupted speech that he is very breathless. On questioning, he tells you that recently he has needed his inhaler much more regularly. In fact he has used 'at least six double doses per day for the past week . . . more today'.

What issues you should cover in management of an episode of acute asthma

In addition to the history obtained, important initial assessment includes:

- symptoms and response to treatment
- peak expiratory flow rate (PEFR)
- respiratory rate (breathing frequency, *see* above)
- pulse rate.

If he has a pyrexia, both breathing frequency and pulse will be raised, making the signs less useful in the evaluation of the severity of the airways obstruction.

Case study 4.2 continued

You examine Mr Dram. His peak flow rate is 250 l/min (his predicted PEFR for his age and height is 620 l/min; the best PEFR recorded in his medical notes was 560 l/min recorded three years ago). His pulse rate is 115 beats per minute, his breathing frequency is 27 breaths per minute and on auscultation, air entry is reduced with a tight expiratory wheeze.

Mr Dram's current PEFR is 45% of his best. This measurement plus your findings on examination are consistent with a diagnosis of acute severe asthma.[1] Assessment should result in a classification of the severity of the asthma:

- *moderate exacerbation*:
  - increasing symptoms
  - PEFR more than 50–75% of the best or predicted
  - no features of severe asthma
- *acute severe*, any one of:
  - inability to complete sentences in one breath
  - PEFR 33–50% of the best or predicted
  - breathing frequency of 25/min or more
  - heart rate of 110/min or more

- *life-threatening*, any one of:
  - silent chest
  - cyanosis
  - feeble respiratory effort
  - slow or irregular pulse or hypotension
  - exhaustion, confusion, coma
  - PEFR less than 33% best or predicted.

Treatment of acute asthma

Oxygen

- Give high flow oxygen.
- Nebulised beta$_2$-agonist bronchodilators should be driven by oxygen.
- If oxygen is not available, give nebulised therapy if indicated.

Steroid therapy

- Give systemic steroids in adequate doses.
- Continue prednisolone 40–50 mg daily for at least five days or until recovery.

Beta$_2$-agonist bronchodilators

- Give high-dose inhaled beta$_2$-agonists as first-line agents as soon as possible via a spacer or nebuliser.
- A nebuliser driven by oxygen is preferable if the asthma is life-threatening.
- Consider continuous nebulised treatment if not responsive to the initial dose.

Other therapies

- Nebulised ipratropium bromide 0.5 mg 4–6 hourly should be added to beta$_2$-agonist in acute severe or life-threatening asthma, or if there is a poor response to beta$_2$-agonist.
- Refer as an emergency to secondary care if not responding or if the attack is life-threatening, for consideration of magnesium sulphate treatment and other supportive therapy, such as mechanical ventilation.

Case study 4.2 continued

You start treatment with oxygen at 40–60% flow rate. You give Mr Dram 5 mg of salbutamol via an oxygen-driven nebuliser. You give him an oral dose of 50 mg of prednisolone immediately. You reassess Mr Dram after 15 minutes. His PEFR has increased to 270 l/min. His pulse rate is 110/minute.

On the basis of his presentation and your knowledge of the patient, you decide that hospital admission is appropriate. You arrange an emergency ambulance to collect Mr Dram from the surgery. You notify the hospital by

---

telephone and provide an admission letter detailing his history, your assessment, and times and types of treatment you have already given. You stay with Mr Dram until the ambulance arrives. You inform the paramedics of the details of presentation, assessment and treatment already given. You advise the paramedics that the patient may require further nebulised beta$_2$-agonists in the ambulance.

Some days later . . .

Mr Dram spends three days in hospital before being discharged. You invite him by telephone to attend for an asthma review. You agree an appointment with the practice nurse, scheduled for the next day.

Follow-up of hospital admission for acute asthma episode

Your plan should be to:

- document the medication being used by Mr Dram
- ask about current and recent symptoms:
  - wheeze
  - tightness of chest
  - shortness of breath
  - cough
  - any provoking factors
  - worsening of symptoms at night
  - frequency of using 'reliever' inhaler
- measure and record his PEFR
- check his inhaler technique.

Agree a written asthma action plan and how it will be implemented with Mr Dram. Arrange and encourage follow-up.

There is a possibility that Mr Dram will not wish to attend for follow-up of his asthma. As healthcare professionals we can only do our best to ensure that should Mr Dram make the decision not to attend for review of his asthma management, he is at least making it as an informed choice.[7]

Quality indicators in asthma

Some of the quality indicators (e.g. smoking status, smoking cessation advice and influenza immunisation) will obviously overlap with those for other areas. Ensure that patients who have not been prescribed asthma-related medication in the last 12 months are removed from the asthma register. Record any other reasons for exclusion, e.g. a serious other illness or inability to perform peak flow or spirometry. The indicators are summarised in Table 4.1.[6]

Table 4.1:   Quality indicators in asthma

Indicator		Points	Maximum threshold (%)
Asthma 1	Register of patients with asthma (excluding those who have not been prescribed asthma-related drugs in the last 12 months).	7	
Asthma 2	Percentage of patients aged eight years and over who have been diagnosed as having asthma from 1 April 2003 and have had the diagnosis confirmed by spirometry or peak flow measurement.	15	70
Asthma 3	Percentage of patients with asthma between the ages of 14 and 19 years who have a record of smoking status in the previous 15 months.	6	70
Asthma 4	Percentage of patients aged 20 years and over with asthma who have a record of smoking status in the past 15 months, except those who have never smoked, where smoking status has been recorded at least once.	6	70
Asthma 5	Percentage of patients with asthma who smoke who have a record that smoking cessation advice or referral to a specialist service, if available, has been offered within the last 15 months.	6	70
Asthma 6	Percentage of patients with asthma who have had an asthma review in the last 15 months.	20	70
Asthma 7	Percentage of patients aged 16 years and over with asthma who have had influenza immunisation in the preceding 1 September to 31 March.	12	70

All minimum thresholds are 25%

Collecting data to demonstrate your learning, competence, performance and standards of service delivery

Example cycle of evidence 4.1

- Focus: clinical care
- Other relevant foci: relationships with patients; treatment in emergencies

Stages of the evidence cycle

Stage 1
Select targets

Stage 2
Set standards

Stage 5
Document it all

Stage 3A/B
Identify needs

Stage 4
Learning/action plan

Case study 4.3

You receive a request for an urgent house call to Mr Gasping. Mr Gasping is 24 years old and has been asthmatic since he was seven years old. His repeat prescription is for a salbutamol MDI as required and beclometasone 200 µg MDI, two puffs twice daily. The request for a visit is made by his partner as Mr Gasping is too short of breath to speak on the phone, and too breathless to travel to surgery. His asthma has been 'going off' for the past few days.

You recognise this as an emergency and arrange for a paramedic ambulance to attend as a 999 call. You set out immediately and arrive at the patient's home as the paramedics do. Mr Gasping is in the midst of an attack of acute severe asthma. After commencing treatment at home with salbutamol 5 mg via an oxygen-driven nebuliser, and intravenous hydrocortisone 200 mg, Mr Gasping is transferred to hospital on 60% oxygen.

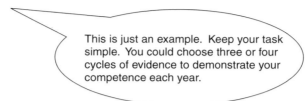

This is just an example. Keep your task simple. You could choose three or four cycles of evidence to demonstrate your competence each year.

Stage 1: Select your aspirations for good practice

The excellent GP:

- has a structured approach for managing long-term health problems and preventive care
- records appropriate information for all contacts including telephone consultations
- responds rapidly to emergencies
- works effectively with the emergency services
- gives patients the information they need about their problems in a way they can understand.

Stage 2: Set the standards for your outcomes

Outcomes might include:

- the way learning is applied
- a learnt skill
- a protocol
- a strategy that is implemented
- meeting recommended standards.

- A consistent, structured approach in the management of asthma.
- The appropriate response of the practice team to emergency situations – with particular reference to asthma.
- A patient-held written asthma action plan is usually agreed.
- The practice recognises the urgent nature of acute severe asthma and responds appropriately.

Stage 3A: Identify your learning needs

- Audit the next 10 patients who consult you with asthma. Establish whether your management appears structured and consistent by comparing against best practice.[1] Identify any gaps in your knowledge or skills.

- Reflect as to whether you feel confident in your abilities to recognise and manage acute severe asthma and are familiar with patient-held written asthma plans.

Stage 3B: Identify your service needs

Any of the needs assessment exercises in 3A may also reveal service needs.

- Review any practice guidelines for the management of asthma and audit the extent to which practice guidelines are applied on 20 patients with asthma randomly selected from the practice register. Identify any problems in its application.
- Audit a further sample of patients (e.g. 20) from your asthma register. Establish how many have been reviewed in the last 15 months. Establish the percentage who have had (i) peak flow rate and recent smoking status recorded, (ii) a peak flow meter prescribed.
- Establish whether your practice promotes the use of personalised asthma diaries and asthma action plans. Find out from 20 consecutive patients attending the asthma review clinic, or 'ordinary' surgeries, the percentage of people with asthma using them.
- Undertake an educational review in your practice to establish whether your reception staff can all recognise a case of acute severe asthma e.g. by discussing fictitious case scenarios.
- Organise a significant event audit of Mr Gasping's case.

Stage 4: Make and carry out a learning and action plan

- Plan an educational programme to suit your learning needs, learning style and what is available. You might attend a lecture or course on asthma, a workshop asthma study day at the local postgraduate centre, use an internet-based learning programme, read books, journals or carry out internet-based research.
- Observe outpatient or general practice-based asthma clinics.
- Arrange a talk at your practice by a local respiratory medicine consultant and/or specialist asthma nurse.
- Arrange a meeting of GPs, nurses and practice managers to discuss and agree the overall structure in which asthma services are delivered.
- Arrange a practice team meeting involving receptionists, practice nurses and doctors for an educational session. Discuss significant event analysis, practice services for asthma, knowledge of asthma, dealing with patients

with asthma and the team's attitude to asthma and pay special consideration to the potentially serious consequences of an asthma attack.

Stage 5: Document your learning, competence, performance and standards of service delivery

- Document all the above processes, including how learning needs and service development needs were arrived at, the course, clinics and other educational events you have participated in, and a record of a workshop run by a local respiratory physician for medical and nursing staff.
- Include the audit of patients on your practice's asthma register, e.g. 50% have a record of peak flow and smoking status, 40% carry personal asthma diaries and action plans.
- Repeat the audit after nine months on patients with asthma described above, showing significant improvement in all criteria audited and fewer presentations of acute severe asthma requiring hospitalisation.
- Keep a log of your visit to a nearby practice with an excellent reputation for the management of asthma and a record of key changes to the organisation of your own practice as a result.
- Include the record of staff baseline knowledge and skills when presented with fictitious cases of asthma and the subsequent practice-based asthma training afternoon for all practice staff on asthma management.

Case study 4.3 continued

You make Mr Gasping's hospital admission the topic of the practice's next significant event audit. You conclude that on the positive side, the urgent nature of Mr Gasping's asthma attack was recognised by both reception and medical staff and appropriate actions were taken. On the negative side, despite being seen with asthma twice over the past year, the last PEFR recorded for Mr Gasping was over two years ago. There was no record of Mr Gasping's smoking status. Analysis of Mr Gasping's repeat prescription requests indicates that his demand for salbutamol inhalers had doubled over the past three months. This had not been sufficient to signal the impending problem on the computerised prescription monitoring system that your practice has in place. On the basis of this, you decide as a practice team to review your practice management of asthma.

Example cycle of evidence 4.2

- Focus: making effective use of resources
- Other relevant focus: good clinical care

Stages of the evidence cycle

Stage 1
Select targets

Stage 2
Set standards

Stage 5
Document it all

Stage 3A/B
Identify needs

Stage 4
Learning/action plan

Case study 4.4

Your practice manager calls a meeting to discuss how to maximise the practice's quality points under the new GMS contract. As lead partner in the management of asthma you are aiming for the quality points for a high 'percentage of patients aged eight years and over diagnosed as having asthma where the diagnosis has been confirmed by spirometry or peak flow measurement'.[6]

That same afternoon Mr Fit, a 19-year-old man, attends for advice. He wishes to join the army and is concerned that he is on the asthma register. He has been told that this may cause problems if he goes to sign up. He was prescribed a salbutamol inhaler some five years ago when he presented with a chest infection. He tells you that he has never needed to use it and on questioning gives no history suggestive of asthma. You can find no evidence of peak flow readings in Mr Fit's notes and there is no objective evidence that he has asthma.

You appreciate from this case that accuracy in diagnosing asthma is an appropriate topic for demonstration of your clinical competence. You decide, as lead asthma partner, to ensure that, where possible, asthma is only diagnosed on the basis of objective evidence.

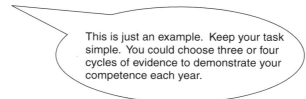

This is just an example. Keep your task simple. You could choose three or four cycles of evidence to demonstrate your competence each year.

Stage 1: Select your aspirations for good practice

The excellent GP:

- makes sound management decisions that are based on good practice and evidence
- uses investigations when they will help with management of the condition
- only prescribes treatments that make an effective contribution to the patient's overall management.

Stage 2: Set the standards for your outcomes

Outcomes might include:

- the way learning is applied
- a learnt skill
- a protocol
- a strategy that is implemented
- meeting recommended standards.

- Every new diagnosis of asthma made in a patient aged eight years and over has been done on the basis of peak flow measurement.

Stage 3A: Identify your learning needs

- Reflect on whether you are putting the criteria for the diagnosis of asthma into practice (look back at Box 4.2, page 58).
- Audit your ability to teach patients to correctly measure and record their own peak flow readings. Seek feedback from the practice nurse about patients' techniques and skills, when he/she is seeing patients you have taught, for follow up at a subsequent practice asthma clinic.

Stage 3B: Identify your service needs

Any of the needs assessment exercises in 3A may also reveal service needs.

- Audit a sample of patients (e.g. 30 to 50) aged eight years or over, who have been put on your practice's asthma register. Establish the percentage that has been diagnosed as having asthma on the basis of peak flow measurements. Establish which health professionals in your primary healthcare team carry out reversibility testing and exercise testing of peak flow rates. Compare all the health professionals involved to see who follows the agreed procedures.
- Audit the next 10 patients who require instruction on peak flow measurement to ensure that they have understood that while standing they should take a deep breath, then blow into the peak flow meter as hard and as fast as they are able.
- Follow individual cases in your sample and review the organisation and procedures followed when performing peak flow measurements, reversibility testing and exercise testing of peak flow – matched against agreed best practice.
- Reflect as to whether there are sufficient and long enough appointments available to allow diagnostic peak flow testing to be done.
- Find out if enough peak flow meters are available for the practice to lend to patients who are asked to monitor their peak flow rates at home for diagnostic purposes. Ask your GP colleagues what they do – does the practice lend patients peak flow meters or are they prescribed?
- Put asthma on the agenda of your practice's next multidisciplinary clinical meeting to see if informal discussion reveals a need for a uniform policy in the diagnosis of asthma.
- Undertake a significant event audit to establish whether the systems for diagnosing asthma in children aged over eight years and adults are in place in your practice, and if they work effectively and efficiently on the basis of peak flow measurements.

Stage 4: Make and carry out a learning and action plan

- Participate in an educational event focused on the diagnosis of asthma. This may be a clinical meeting, sitting in on a consultant or asthma nurse specialist meeting or any other educational event.
- Re-read the criteria for the diagnosis of asthma in the British guidelines on the management of asthma.[1–3]

- Encourage other members of the primary care team involved in diagnosing asthma to participate in education.
- Organise a practice meeting to share best practice in diagnosing asthma and involve your partners, nurses, staff and practice manager in the organisational restructuring necessary to ensure that peak flow testing is readily available to possible new asthma patients.

Stage 5 Document your learning, competence, performance and standards of service delivery

- Document all the work and meetings undertaken above.
- Record the regular audits to establish the percentage of newly diagnosed asthmatic patients in whom diagnosis is based on peak flow measurements, for all members of the team.
- Record the monitoring of the availability of appointments for reversibility testing.

Case study 4.4 continued

You review Mr Fit's case, and review his current peak flow diary, then remove him from the practice's asthma register.

Your audits demonstrate that your patients have learnt how to measure peak flow correctly. The team agrees a practice guideline on the diagnosis of asthma in patients aged eight years and over, based on what they have learnt and the British guidelines on the management of asthma.[1] You also discuss the availability of the clinical time required to correctly manage asthma with your practice manager and nursing staff.

After six months, a repeat audit of patients aged eight years and over who have been placed on the asthma register in the past six months shows that for 97% of them this has been on the basis of diagnostically significant variance in peak flow measurement. You claim maximum points for this area from the quality and outcomes framework.

Example cycle of evidence 4.3

- Focus: clinical care
- Other relevant focus: making effective use of resources

Stages of the evidence cycle

Stage 1
Select targets

Stage 2
Set standards

Stage 5
Document it all

Stage 3A/B
Identify needs

Stage 4
Learning/action plan

Case study 4.5

You are asked to visit Mr Vent, a 46-year-old known to have asthma. Although the reason for the house call is unrelated to his asthma, you cannot help but notice a line of seven salbutamol inhalers on his bedside table. He tells you that he never seems to need to use his salbutamol. He is however on a high dose of inhaled steroid and a long-acting beta$_2$-agonist.

You ask Mr Vent to attend the practice's asthma clinic for an asthma review. You suspect that it would be appropriate to step down his treatment. You decide to take a closer look at the practice asthma clinic protocol, including criteria for stepping up and stepping down patients' treatment.

This is just an example. Keep your task simple. You could choose three or four cycles of evidence to demonstrate your competence each year.

Stage 1: Select your aspirations for good practice

The excellent GP:

- has a structured approach for managing long-term health problems
- only prescribes treatments that make an effective contribution to the patient's overall management.

Stage 2: Set the standards for your outcomes

Outcomes might include:

- the way learning is applied
- a learnt skill
- a protocol
- a strategy that is implemented
- meeting recommended standards.

- The call and recall system used by your practice's asthma clinic operates to ensure that all patients on your asthma register are invited to attend regularly.
- Appropriate information is collected and an examination is performed at your practice's asthma clinic in line with the best practice protocol.[1]
- It can be demonstrated in a random sample of patients that an individual asthmatic's treatment is always stepped up and stepped down as that patient's condition dictates.

Stage 3A: Identify your learning needs

- Reflect whether you are aware of the history and examination findings that should be recorded during an asthma clinic review.
- Ask others in the team to give you feedback about how well you apply the criteria to step up or step down a patient's asthma treatment e.g. ask the local pharmacist, the practice nurse running the practice asthma clinic, etc.

Stage 3B: Identify your service needs

Any of the needs assessment exercises in 3A may also reveal service needs.

- Summarise the system your practice uses to arrange call and recall to your asthma clinic. Establish how information is collected at the asthma clinic –

by computer or paper template and what written guidelines there are. Compare with the systems and information in another general practice recognised as leading on asthma management in your PCO.

- Audit patients' attendance rate at the asthma clinic and consider if the recall system and timing of asthma clinics could be redesigned to improve rates.
- Review the system used by your practice to amend a patient's asthma medication prescription when treatment is stepped up or stepped down.
- Undertake a SWOT analysis (*see* page 24) of asthma management services in the practice. Feed in the results of audits and reviews, including whether patient data collected at the asthma clinic is complete according to the practice protocol. If data is incomplete, establish why.
- Identify any training needs in the nursing and other staff involved in the running of your asthma clinic.

Stage 4: Make and carry out a learning and action plan

- Learn from written material, for example reviewing national guidelines,[1] and/or sit in on an asthma clinic, visit another practice, attend lectures or undertake internet-based educational programmes.
- Discuss and agree a practice asthma clinic guideline with the partners and nursing staff at your practice.
- Hold a practice meeting to agree aspects of practice and asthma clinic organisation, and allocate sufficient resources to meet the quality and outcomes you have set out in your practice protocol. This should include well co-ordinated systems as well as doctor time, nurse time, administrative staff time, practical equipment and information aids for patients.
- Organise an educational programme in the practice to meet any staff training needs that you have identified, or arrange training elsewhere.

Stage 5: Document your learning, competence, performance and standards of service delivery

- Document the work undertaken as described in the stages above as a semi-formal review of your performance and the performance of your practice against the outcomes you have set.
- Include a copy of national guidelines on the management of asthma.[1]
- Record your visit to an asthma clinic run by a practice known to take a special interest in respiratory disease.
- Include your notes from discussion with one of the local asthma nurses about her recommended criteria for the 'ideal' asthma clinic.
- Keep copies of the audits undertaken (*see* above).

- Include your notes from a practice meeting with GPs, practice nurses, the practice manager and yourself, attended by a local respiratory consultant and respiratory nurse. Keep a copy of the resulting new practice asthma protocol that includes an emphasis on stepping up and stepping down asthma treatment as appropriate.

Case study 4.5 continued

Six months later, you repeat your audit of both the percentage of patients who have attended for an asthma review and the data recorded about these patients. You find significant improvements in both criteria. From examination of the records of patients on the asthma register, you also find examples of appropriate stepping up and stepping down of asthma treatment.

    You step Mr Vent's treatment down and the practice nurse follows him up at a successive appointment in the asthma review clinic. Six months later, he is maintained at Step 2 of regular preventive therapy with a low dose of inhaled steroid only.

References

1 Foord-Kelcey G (ed.) (2003) British guideline on the management of asthma in adults. *Guidelines.* **21:** 113–15.

2 Thiadens HA, de Bock GH and Dekker FW *et al.* (1988) Identifying asthma and chronic obstructive pulmonary disease in patients with persistent cough presenting to general practitioners: descriptive study. *British Medical Journal.* **316:** 1286–90.

3 The British Thoracic Society, 17 Doughty Street, London EC1N 2PL and www.brit-thoracic.org.uk Guidelines at www.brit-thoracic.org.uk/sign/index.htm

4 Scottish Intercollegiate Guidelines Network (SIGN), Royal College of Physicians, 9 Queen Street, Edinburgh EH2 1JQ and www.sign.ac.uk

5 National Asthma Campaign www.asthma.org.uk

6 General Practitioners Committee/The NHS Confederation (2003) *New GMS Contract 2003. Investing in general practice.* General Practitioners' Committee/ NHS Confederation, London.

7 Royal College of General Practitioners/General Practitioners Committee (2002) *Good Medical Practice for General Practitioners.* Royal College of General Practitioners, London.

5

Chronic obstructive pulmonary disease

Case study 5.1

Mr Hough is a 50-year-old who runs a small and ramshackle sheep farm. He attends in the autumn complaining that he has already seen 'that young doctor' and has had two lots of antibiotics without effect. He has come back about the X-ray that the GP registrar arranged and wants you to give him some strong antibiotics to 'clear it up', like he usually has each winter. The chest X-ray is clear.

   You go over his history again and hear that he always has a cough but it has worsened. He is finding it difficult to do his work because he gets so out of breath. He has smoked for years but has always blamed the dust at the farm for his cough that is present daily and worse in the mornings. Examination does not make things much clearer and the peak flow test does not tell you much apart from his lack of ability to blow down the mouthpiece. You tell him that you think he may have chronic obstructive pulmonary disease (COPD) and that you will arrange some tests. You arrange these as soon as you can, as Mr Hough is obviously displeased with your response to his request for antibiotics, despite acknowledging that they haven't done much good so far. You suggest he continues with the inhaler he has used intermittently for some years, and arrange to check his technique when he attends next. You explain about the tests he needs and give him the information sheet for his spirometry testing, so that he knows when to stop his treatment before the tests.

What issues you should cover

Like Mr Hough, most people are poorly informed about COPD. In a MORI poll, only one in three members of the public had heard of COPD, but many more recognised the terms chronic bronchitis and emphysema.[1] Few of those interviewed were aware that COPD is common and is mainly caused by smoking. Many people experience persistent respiratory symptoms but only just over half of the respondents suggested that breathlessness on exertion or coughing could be the first signs of a serious lung disease. In two out of three people with symptoms, this was because they were unconcerned or unaware that their symptoms could be important, and in nearly one in four cases this was because they thought they would simply be told to stop smoking.

COPD is a major cause of death and disability.[2] In your PCO there are likely to be 54–55 deaths from COPD each year (compared with only 2–3 deaths from asthma). Up to 25% of deaths from COPD occur before retirement age. By 2020, COPD is forecast to become the fifth most frequent cause of death.[3] In the UK, as many as one in eight medical admissions are due to COPD and emergency admissions have risen dramatically recently, especially in early January.[4]

The prevalence of COPD is greatest in socio-economically deprived people. The underlying cause is unknown and still under investigation. Genetic susceptibility to the disease is also being studied. Diagnosis is based on the history together with spirometry.

A definition of COPD[5]

COPD is a disease state characterised by airflow limitation that is not fully reversible. Airflow limitation is usually progressive and associated with an abnormal inflammatory response of the lungs to irritation. The symptoms are usually cough, production of sputum and breathlessness on exertion. Episodes of sudden worsening of the symptoms often occur. Other diagnostic labels included in COPD include:

- chronic bronchitis
- emphysema
- chronic obstructive airways disease
- chronic airways limitation
- some cases of chronic asthma.

Asthma shows reversible airflow limitation, although some chronic asthma may blur into COPD when reversibility is not complete. Chronic bronchitis is defined as the presence of cough and sputum production for at least three months in each of two consecutive years, not necessarily with airflow limitation. Emphysema, defined as the destruction of the alveoli, is a pathological term but is often used loosely as a clinical diagnosis.

Clinical features

Symptoms

Cigarette or other types of tobacco smoking is the main risk factor for COPD. Other causes of COPD may include:

- occupational dust and chemicals (vapours, irritants and fumes) when exposure is prolonged or intense
- indoor air pollution from biomass fuel (wood, dung, etc) used for cooking and heating in poorly ventilated dwellings
- outdoor air pollution.

NICE guidance recommends that GPs consider a diagnosis of COPD in smokers over the age of 35 years who present with breathlessness on exertion, chronic cough, regular sputum production, frequent bronchitis or wheeze.[6]

Mr Hough may be right that dust contributes to his chronic cough, but it is likely that his cigarette habit is the main cause. He has the two main symptoms – shortness of breath and cough. He has also had recurrent infections each winter. If he had large amounts of sputum, you might consider a diagnosis of bronchiectasis. Ask about coughing up blood. This is usually due to infection, but could suggest cancer of the bronchus and would prompt an immediate referral for secondary care investigation.

Mr Hough's breathlessness at present is probably following an infective episode, but he may not have realised how short of breath he was becoming until it suddenly became worse. The breathlessness increases gradually over several years until it becomes obvious. Like many sufferers, Mr Hough has had wheezing with his infective episodes in the past and has been prescribed a bronchodilator inhaler.

Patients who have long-standing disease with emphysema (previously known as 'pink puffers') may have considerable weight loss. Those with chronic hypoxia leading to cor pulmonale (previously known as 'blue bloaters') tend to gain weight. The two old-fashioned descriptive categories are not useful for management.

Examination

As in Mr Hough's case, examination is rarely helpful. You may think of emphysema if the chest is barrel shaped with reduced expansion and the breathing is laboured with pursed lips and use of the accessory respiratory muscles.

In advanced disease, peripheral oedema, raised jugular venous pressure, hepatic congestion and a flapping tremor may suggest cor pulmonale.

Other diagnoses to consider for complaints of cough and breathlessness

The main confusion is with chronic asthma. The main features that differentiate COPD from other conditions appear in Table 5.1.

Table 5.1: Differential diagnosis of cough and breathlessness

Diagnosis	Symptoms	Signs	Chest X-ray	Lung function
COPD	Mid-life, slow onset; exposure to tobacco smoke	Usually none in the early stages	Normal or may show emphysema	Airflow limitation mostly irreversible
Asthma	Early life, often childhood; variable day to day; allergy, rhinitis, eczema often also present; family history	None or expiratory wheeze	Normal	Airflow limitation mostly reversible
Congestive heart failure	Mid to later life; history of heart disease	Fine crackles at lung bases	Dilated heart; pulmonary oedema	Volume restriction, not airflow limitation
Tuberculosis	Any age; history of contact or from an area of prevalence	None or signs of infection	Lung infiltrate or nodular lesions	Not applicable; microbiological confirmation needed

Spirometry

Spirometry uses a spirometer to measure how effectively and how quickly an individual can breathe out to empty the lungs. The curve measured is called the spirogram and measures volume against time. A booklet on spirometry can be downloaded from the British Thoracic Society website as well as several other useful information booklets on COPD.[7]

Practices will vary in how they arrange for spirometry tests. NICE guidelines recommend that all healthcare professionals caring for patients with COPD should have access to spirometry and know how to interpret the results.[6] Some practices will purchase a spirometer and have practice nurses who have been trained in performing and interpreting the tests. The equipment is not expensive but the tests are time consuming and take practice nurses away from other duties for a considerable time. Most patients will need at least a 30-minute appointment and the equipment needs cleaning, calibrating and maintaining. Some practices refer to a service provided by the PCO on a locality basis, either by in-house provision or by an outreach provision from the hospital trust. In other areas, the hospital trust provides an open-access service.

Patients are usually anxious about the test, so spending a little time recording how their life is affected by their symptoms is useful as a baseline and can help to settle them down. Explain the test carefully – a demonstration helps. The test is not affected by whether the patient sits or stands, so most patients sit in case they feel dizzy performing the tests. The patient:

- takes a deep breath in
- seals the lips around the mouthpiece
- forces the air out of the chest as hard and as fast as they can until the lungs feel empty
- breathes in again and relaxes.

Patients occasionally need a nose clip to help them breathe out through the mouth. Repeat the readings until three curves are within 100 ml or 5% of each other and therefore reproducible. Breathing out must be for at least 6 seconds and can take up to 15 seconds. Some patients find the test impossible to do, despite much encouragement, especially if they have a frequent cough or chest pain.

The spirometer may print out the results or display them on a screen. Spirometry measures:

- forced vital capacity (FVC)
- forced expiratory volume in one second (FEV_1).

The results are compared with the 'percentage predicted' using the appropriate normal values for an individual's age, sex and height. Typically, a patient with COPD shows a decrease in FEV_1 and in the percentage FEV_1/FVC. The European guidelines define three stages of severity, based on the measured FEV_1 as a percentage of the predicted FEV_1:[8]

- FEV_1 more than or equal to 70% predicted: **mild**
- FEV_1 between 50–69% predicted: **moderate**
- FEV_1 less than 50% predicted: **severe**.

You will usually need to do reversibility testing as well (*see* Table 5.2; *see* also Chapter 4 on asthma).

Many patients in the mild and moderate European stages do not present with symptoms. A more useful classification for deciding on treatment appears in the guidelines from the Global Initiative for Chronic Obstructive Lung Disease[9] (*see* Table 5.3, page 88).

Table 5.2:   Reversibility testing[10]

Bronchodilator	Dose	FEV_1 before and after
Salbutamol	2.5–5 mg (nebuliser) 200–400 µg (large-volume spacer)	15 min
Terbutaline	5–10 mg (nebuliser) 500 µg (large-volume spacer)	15 min
Ipratropium bromide	500 µg (nebuliser) 160 µg large-volume spacer	30 min

Steroid
  Prednisolone
  Beclometasone dipropionate/
    budesonide
	30 mg/day (oral)
	
	1000 µg/day (large-volume spacer)
		2 weeks
		
		6 weeks

Fluticasone proprionate	500 µg/day (large-volume spacer)	6 weeks

Management of chronic obstructive pulmonary disease

Smoking cessation

This is an ideal time to tackle Mr Hough's smoking habit.[11] He will be more receptive while he has symptoms. Tell him about the damage he is doing to his lungs and explain that stopping smoking is probably the most effective way of preventing the progression of his lung disease. Warn him that when he stops smoking he may have withdrawal symptoms. These may include irritability or aggression, depression, restlessness, impaired concentration, increased appetite and craving for cigarettes. Mr Hough may also experience light-headedness and disturbed sleep.

Psychological and behavioural techniques are key to helping patients to stop smoking. People trained in supporting smoking cessation acquire skills to maintain motivation and appreciate the underlying psychology of addiction and withdrawal. You may be able to refer Mr Hough to a smoking cessation service that will assess what techniques would help him most and give him support while he quits. Combining psychological and behavioural counselling, or group support with pharmacological interventions such as nicotine replacement or bupropion therapy, increases smoking cessation rates. Using these combination therapies, nearly one in five are still ex-smokers at six months after stopping smoking. However, longer-term follow-up studies show that many ex-smokers relapse and start smoking again.[11] Indicate your willingness to prescribe nicotine replacement therapy for Mr Hough.

Some patients find acupuncture and hypnotherapy helpful although there is little research evidence about their effectiveness. Smoking is a coping mechanism for many smokers who believe that cigarettes calm them down if they are worried or anxious. Many smokers will have tried unsuccessfully to give up in the past – and you will be trying to motivate Mr Hough to quit smoking so anything you can suggest that might make him feel more in control of his smoking may help.

Many health professionals are familiar with the well-known staged approach where patients are assessed for their readiness to change, and smoking cessation interventions are tailored to the stage patients have reached. Conclusions from a systematic review were that, overall, stage-based interventions are no more effective than non-stage-based interventions or no intervention, in changing smoking behaviour.[12]

Exercise training and rehabilitation[13]

Approximately one-third of hospitals in the UK provide rehabilitation courses for people with chronic lung disease, and the majority of these use hospital facilities. Most of the hospital programmes use outpatient programmes and there is limited experience of providing inpatient, home, or community rehabilitation. However, recently the potential for rehabilitation in primary care is beginning to be explored. The courses are run by a multiprofessional team of physiotherapists, dietitians, medical and nursing staff. Most consist of a six-week outpatient programme with two supervised sessions a week and additional instructions to train at home on a daily basis. More intensive inpatient courses are sometimes provided, but are more expensive. The courses include aerobic physical exercise training and information on disease education. Additional components can include limb-strength and upper limb training, psychological and nutritional intervention and, of course, smoking cessation. A comprehensive, individually tailored, programme of rehabilitation will improve functional exercise capacity, reduce exertional dyspnoea, and improve health status.[10] Health economic benefits of rehabilitation are only just beginning to be explored, but reductions in hospital admission frequency, duration of stay, exacerbation rate, GP home visits, and bronchodilator usage have all been reported.[10]

Therapy

The guidelines from the Global Initiative for Chronic Obstructive Lung Disease[7] were updated in 2003 and the new guidelines set out the stages slightly differently from those from 2001. However, treatment options have not changed (*see* Table 5.3).

Table 5.3:   Therapy at each stage of COPD[7]

Stage	Characteristics	Treatment options
All		Avoidance of risk factors Influenza immunisation
Stage 0: At risk	Chronic symptoms Exposure to risk factors Normal spirometry	As above
Stage I: Mild	FEV_1/FVC less than 70% FEV_1 at or more than 80% With or without symptoms	Add short-acting bronchodilator when needed
Stage II: Moderate	FEV_1/FVC less than 70%	Add regular treatment with one or more long-acting bronchodilators
	FEV_1 between 50 and 80% With or without symptoms	Add rehabilitation
Stage III: Severe	FEV_1/FVC less than 70% FEV_1 between 30 and 50% With or without symptoms	Add inhaled corticosteroids if the patient has repeated exacerbations
Stage IV: Very severe	FEV_1/FVC less than 70%	Add long-term oxygen if the patient has respiratory failure
	FEV_1 less than 30% With chronic respiratory failure or cor pulmonale	Consider surgical treatments e.g. bullectomy or lung transplantation

The treatments listed do not include methylxanthines. On the small amount of evidence that has been published, they have not been shown to be particularly effective and can cause considerable harm from side-effects (nausea and vomiting, tremor, palpitations or arrhythmias).[14] Some guidelines still include them, so you should check that your guidelines are up to date and what local specialists recommend.

Mr Hough's symptoms suggest that he is in transition from stage I to stage II, but this should be confirmed with spirometry.

Nebulised drugs are considerably more expensive than other forms of inhaled therapy. Only start long-term nebulised treatment in COPD after a full assessment by a respiratory specialist or GP with specific training. Many patients may achieve similar benefit by using a large-volume spacer with high-dose bronchodilator (up to eight puffs, four times daily). All assessments for nebuliser treatment should include a trial of drug administration via large-volume spacers. Discourage patients from buying their own nebuliser without a proper assessment for long-term treatment.

Referral to secondary care

You might refer Mr Hough to a respiratory clinic at this stage if:

- he needs rehabilitation, the hospital provides this, and no community scheme exists
- you are uncertain of the diagnosis or he wants an expert opinion
- he has other medical conditions complicating his management
- he is more seriously affected than his symptoms suggest.

After referral, he might have full lung function testing, arterial blood gases, exercise testing, computerised tomography (CT) scan and an oral steroid trial.

Some areas have outreach specialist nurses who can help patients with the management of their condition at home, once their diagnosis and treatment has been sorted out.[15]

Management of exacerbations[7]

The severity of an exacerbation can be assessed from the symptoms and by using a peak flow meter (a patient with a severe exacerbation has a reading of less than 100 l/min or a FEV_1 of below 1 l). If the patient is admitted to hospital, arterial blood gases can be used. You may want to do a chest X-ray and electrocardiogram (ECG) to exclude other diagnoses. Sputum culture with sensitivities may be useful.

Management at home includes:

- increasing the dose and/or frequency of the existing bronchodilator
- if not already in use, adding anticholinergic therapy
- if the FEV_1 is less than 50% of that predicted for age, sex and height, adding 40 mg of prednisolone daily for 10 days
- if the sputum is purulent and increased in amount, adding antibiotics according to local patterns of antibiotic sensitivity.

Referral for hospital admission is usually indicated when there is:

- a sudden increase in symptoms
- worsening of severe COPD
- new physical signs such as cyanosis or peripheral oedema
- failure to respond to therapy
- significant other medical conditions
- uncertainty about the diagnosis
- insufficient home support.

Organising continuing care

Making the diagnosis, educating the patient, arranging for exercise and rehabilitation and initiating treatment are only the first steps in managing this chronic condition. Mr Hough will need regular review, probably annually. This will meet your quality indicators (*see* below) and provide proactive management to try to avoid sudden decompensation. Making a practice nurse and doctor combination responsible for this domain is a sensible arrangement in a group practice, but may require co-operation with other practices, or provision by the PCO for smaller or single-handed practices. The current guidelines will help with deciding what to cover at each review but you might want to consider:

- symptom assessment
- smoking status and smoking cessation advice if required
- inhaler use and technique (patients need a large-volume spacer)
- spirometry
- measurement of oxygen saturation with a finger probe pulse oximeter
- advice about influenza immunisations if required
- advice about pneumococcal immunisation
- support and encouragement about diet, exercise and daily living activities.

Quality indicators in chronic obstructive pulmonary disease

As with asthma in Chapter 4, some of the quality indicators (smoking status and smoking cessation advice) will overlap with those for other areas. The indicators are summarised in Table 5.4.

Unfortunately because of the confusion about the stages of severity, drawing up the register will be the most difficult part. The contract specifies a definition of COPD as:

- FEV_1 less than 70% of that predicted for age, sex and height
- FEV_1 /FVC ratio less than 70%
- reversibility less than 15%.

There will be patients who are somewhere in that blurred area between chronic asthma and COPD. If they do not fall into the categories listed above they may need to be classified on the asthma register, although their management may be more like that of someone with COPD!

Table 5.4: Quality indicators in chronic obstructive pulmonary disease

Indicator		Points	Maximum threshold (%)
COPD 1	A register of patients with COPD.	5	
COPD 2	Percentage of patients with a new diagnosis of COPD since April 2003 confirmed by spirometry and reversibility testing.	5	90
COPD 3	Percentage of patients on the COPD register who have had their diagnosis confirmed by spirometry and reversibility testing.	5	90
COPD 4	Percentage of patients on the COPD register who have had their smoking status recorded in the last 15 months.	6	90
COPD 5	Percentage of patients on the COPD register who smoke and who have been offered smoking cessation advice in the last 15 months.	6	90
COPD 6	Percentage of patients on the COPD register who have had their FEV_1 recorded in the previous 27 months.	6	70
COPD 7	Percentage of patients on the COPD register who have had their inhaler technique checked in the previous 2 years.	6	90
COPD 8	Percentage of patients on the COPD register who have had an influenza immunisation in the preceding 1 September to 31 March.	7	85

All minimum thresholds are 25%

Collecting data to demonstrate your learning, competence, performance and standards of service delivery

Example cycle of evidence 5.1

- Focus: clinical care
- Other relevant foci: working with colleagues; relationships with patients; probity

Stages of the evidence cycle

Stage 1
Select targets

Stage 2
Set standards

Stage 5
Document it all

Stage 3A/B
Identify needs

Stage 4
Learning/action plan

Case study 5.2

Dr Truly is lead clinician for asthma and COPD in her practice. The practice already has a disease register for asthma but as she and the practice nurse go through the records, they find that quite a few people should be classified as having COPD. She is concerned that the quality points that the practice think that they should be able to gain cannot be demonstrated by the data. She finds that evidence about non-smokers is easy to demonstrate, as it only needs to be recorded once. However, many of the records about current smoking are out of date and do not indicate whether smokers are receiving advice or have had their status checked.

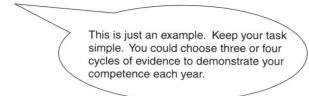

This is just an example. Keep your task simple. You could choose three or four cycles of evidence to demonstrate your competence each year.

Stage 1: Select your aspirations for good practice

The excellent GP:

- makes and records accurate diagnoses in patients' medical records
- plays his/her part in maintaining recording systems of chronic disease management in the practice.

Stage 2: Set the standards for your outcomes

Outcomes might include:

- the way learning is applied
- a learnt skill
- a protocol
- a strategy that is implemented
- meeting recommended standards.

- Every patient on the disease register for COPD has a record of the spirometry readings confirming the diagnosis.
- There is a structured approach for managing long-term health problems and preventive care.
- All patients on regular review for long-term health problems have a record of their smoking status and have been given smoking cessation advice if relevant.

Stage 3A: Identify your learning needs

- Self-assess your knowledge of the diagnostic criteria for COPD.
- Carry out a patient survey: ask 10 consecutive patients who smoke (some of whom should be on the COPD register) if they have received advice about smoking within the previous two years, and if so, how appropriate the advice was perceived to be, when it had been given and by whom.

Stage 3B: Identify your service needs

> Any of the needs assessment exercises in 3A may also reveal service needs.

- Audit the smoking status of patients on the COPD register for the existence of records of smoking status in the last 12 months, the extent of advice and support or help offered and the change of smoking behaviour since the last review.
- With colleagues, carry out a force-field analysis of the driving and re-straining forces for the management of long-term health problems such as COPD in your practice.

Stage 4: Make and carry out a learning and action plan

- Read up about the risks of smoking and provision of best practice in motivating people to stop smoking.
- Talk to smokers at an informal group, e.g. in the waiting room during influenza immunisation, and actively listen to their feedback about improving services and the quality and extent of the advice they have received about stopping smoking.
- Attend a refresher course with the practice nurse on the diagnosis and management of COPD.
- Present your findings (audits, patients survey and force-field analysis) at a practice meeting and obtain the support of the practice team for a more proactive approach to COPD. Invite a respiratory nurse (and/or a patient) to attend and give their perspectives.

Stage 5: Document your learning, competence, performance and standards of service delivery

- Re-audit the records of patients on the COPD register to establish whether the diagnostic criteria are being recorded.
- Include a copy of the practice protocol relating to smoking cessation.
- Re-audit the records of patients on the COPD register for smoking status, extent of advice and support or help offered and the number who have changed their smoking behaviour.
- Keep your notes on the informal feedback from smokers about their experiences.
- Include a copy of the development plan made at the practice meeting to provide a more proactive approach to the management of COPD and a date for a review of progress in 12 months.

Case study 5.2 continued

After 12 months, the re-audit shows the results after the changes made. The data now back up the assertion that all new patients on the COPD register had their diagnostic criteria recorded. Dr Truly and the practice nurse are gradually working their way through the patients previously diagnosed as having COPD, to establish that they are correctly categorised. Dr Truly is also pleased to see that the smoking cessation efforts appear to be making small numbers of people who are at risk change their smoking habits. The other GPs are pleased to hear that they can substantiate their claim for quality points.

Example cycle of evidence 5.2

- Focus: relationships with patients
- Other relevant foci: clinical care; working with colleagues

Stages of the evidence cycle

Stage 1
Select targets

Stage 2
Set standards

Stage 3A/B
Identify needs

Stage 4
Learning/action plan

Stage 5
Document it all

Case study 5.3

Mr Coffer was given early retirement because his long-term bronchitis made him unable to continue with his work as a refuse collector. His wife made him an appointment with the practice nurse because she thought he needed a stronger inhaler. He has had a wheezy chest with infections for years but recently has found that he cannot manage the stairs at home without stopping halfway up. The practice nurse has referred Mr Coffer on to you. She has recently been on a course and become accredited in spirometry[10] and is concerned that he has severe COPD. She has asked for him to be assessed for rehabilitation and nebulised therapy. She also mentions a home oxygen concentrator as Mrs Coffer says her husband goes blue when he gets to the top of the stairs. Mr Coffer is sure that it's just old age and seems to expect you to agree with his view that 'that young woman needs her head examined expecting me to be more active at my age'.

This is just an example. Keep your task simple. You could choose three or four cycles of evidence to demonstrate your competence each year.

Stage 1: Select your aspirations for good practice

The excellent GP:

- is up to date with developments in clinical practice and regularly reviews his or her knowledge and performance
- only prescribes treatments that make an effective contribution to the patient's overall management
- accompanies referrals with the information needed by the specialist to make an appropriate and efficient evaluation of the patient's problem
- does not denigrate the contributions of colleagues.

Stage 2: Set the standards for your outcomes

Outcomes might include:

- the way learning is applied
- a learnt skill
- a protocol
- a strategy that is implemented
- meeting recommended standards.

- Practice management guidelines for COPD are agreed.
- An audit of outcomes of patient referrals for COPD, including patients' perspectives, is in line with intended practice.

Stage 3A: Identify your learning needs

- Compare the current practice guidelines with other guidelines[7] and information the practice nurse acquired while she was on the spirometry course.
- Review your knowledge about the indications and the prescribing arrangements for oxygen concentrators.[16]
- Carry out a survey of patients whom you have treated for COPD to determine the extent of their limitations of daily activities.[17] You might identify 10 consecutive patients from your COPD register, or from a search for data on the prescribing of bronchodilators in people over the age of 55 years.
- Carry out a record review of the last five patients referred to the respiratory clinic, to establish whether you had described the limitations of daily living and the aims of the referral.

Stage 3B: Identify your service needs

Any of the needs assessment exercises in 3A may also reveal service needs.

- Audit the repeat prescribing of people over 55 years who are using three or more inhalers, by asking 20 patients to attend for review of their medication. Find out how long it is since the patient was reviewed, the extent of the relief of symptoms, and whether they have had smoking cessation advice and support, rehabilitation and education about their condition.
- Review the length of time patients with COPD are waiting after referral for their first appointment at a respiratory clinic, for the assessment process and for rehabilitation. Consider what you might have done to speed any of these processes including supplying evidence to your PCO to influence the commissioning process.

Stage 4: Make and carry out a learning and action plan

- Ask the local respiratory physician with members of his/her team to present, to a multidisciplinary meeting, what they can do, inviting several local practices to maximise the impact.
- Draw up with the practice nurse a draft best practice management plan for patients with COPD for discussion at a clinical practice meeting, and present this with the results of the patient survey and audits.
- Discuss how the agreed management policy can be implemented with key people in the practice team, including a local pharmacist, and decide what shortfalls there are in terms of resources (e.g. availability of equipment or

therapy or over-long referral routes) and liaise with the PCO about unmet needs.

- Compare your referral letters to the respiratory clinic with those of colleagues and with examples from the literature of best practice. Draw up a template to guide you so that all relevant information is included.

Stage 5: Document your learning, competence, performance and standards of service delivery

- Include the best practice management plan for patients with COPD.
- Record your survey of the extent of patients' limitations of daily living activities.
- Include the data on content of referral letters and the template for future referral letters.
- Include the results of the audit of the repeat prescribing of people over 55 years who are using three or more inhalers.
- Keep a copy of the information on the management of advanced COPD including the information on assessment and prescription of oxygen concentrators.[16,17]
- Keep a copy of the correspondence with the PCO about the shortfalls in provision of treatment for patients with COPD.

Case study 5.3 continued

The PCO used the information you gathered about the inadequacy of resources for prompt management of patients with COPD, to review the effectiveness of the referral pathway. This resulted in investment of additional resources to fund rehabilitation. The practice team thanked the practice nurse for her input into improving best practice in the management of COPD and felt that the investment in her extra training had been worthwhile.

Example cycle of evidence 5.3

- Focus: research
- Other relevant foci: clinical care; working with colleagues

Stages of the evidence cycle

Stage 1
Select targets

Stage 2
Set standards

Stage 5
Document it all

Stage 3A/B
Identify needs

Stage 4
Learning/action plan

Case study 5.4

A new respiratory physician has taken up post at your local university. He has started several research projects. He is actively recruiting patients for his various trials and asks your practice to refer patients to his team. He needs patients with COPD to take part in a trial of using oxygen while doing intensive exercise training, and another for electrically stimulating muscles in chair-bound patients. You can see that patients will benefit from the speedy referral process, but you are worried that patients may be put on oxygen therapy unnecessarily.

This is just an example. Keep your task simple. You could choose three or four cycles of evidence to demonstrate your competence each year.

Stage 1: Select your aspirations for good practice

The excellent GP:

- protects patients' rights and makes sure that they are not disadvantaged by taking part in research
- has information available on laws and requirements (e.g. research ethics) relating to general practice.

Stage 2: Set the standards for your outcomes

Outcomes might include:

- the way learning is applied
- a learnt skill
- a protocol
- a strategy that is implemented
- meeting recommended standards.

- The practice has a policy for GPs and staff undertaking research, in line with research governance guidelines.
- You have library and learning resources for COPD management available.

Stage 3A: Identify your learning needs

- Find out if you can easily access paper-based resources (e.g. books or files) or electronic sites describing best practice in the management of COPD in your practice.
- Reflect on whether you are up to date with current requirements for undertaking research or participating in someone else's research study. Decide if you are clear about research governance, what studies require ethics approval, how you obtain your PCO's permission to host research, what information patients need before giving their consent to participate in research, etc.

Stage 3B: Identify your service needs

Any of the needs assessment exercises in 3A may also reveal service needs.

- Compare best practice in managing COPD with the interventions that the university research team are proposing in their research. Seek an independent view (e.g. another specialist from outside the trial) as to whether patients will be disadvantaged by you referring them to the trial, remembering the benefits of a speedy referral process. Alternatively, you could ask to see any peer review already carried out about the proposed research.

- Ask the PCO for a copy of the algorithm describing research governance management systems and guidance on how they affect you. Discuss with others in the practice what systems you need to develop to link into the new NHS requirements.
- Ask several patients to comment on the trial's patient information leaflet to check that it is suitable for patients in your population.

Stage 4: Make and carry out a learning and action plan

- Meet the research governance manager for a tutorial on research ethics and research governance systems. Compose a policy for practice staff to fit the legal and NHS requirements, defining the boundary between audit and research.
- Write out what constitutes best practice in managing COPD. Then compare previous treatment with the next case of each that presents, and add notes about any subsequent change of treatment.
- Attend a seminar by the university research team introducing their research plans and put specific questions and queries to the team.
- Compile a list of library or other resources (paper or electronic) your practice needs to buy so that there is sufficient reference material available in relation to COPD management and research ethics. Check your choice with your local health librarian if possible and place an order.

Stage 5: Document your learning, competence, performance and standards of service delivery

- Keep a copy of the practice policy on GPs and staff undertaking research.
- List the contents of the reference library in the practice and the resources available in each consulting room e.g. paper and electronic versions of *Clinical Evidence*.[18]
- Include a copy of the research ethics approval and details of the research study in which you intend to participate.
- Record the questions and answers from the research seminar.
- Keep a checklist of best practice in the management of COPD and the evidence that patients do not become dependent on oxygen once started.

Case study 5.4 continued

After your preparations in understanding and preparing for participating in the research study, all goes smoothly. Patients are happy with the information leaflet about the trials and most consent to join in. Nearly all the local GPs and practices co-operate to refer suitable patients so that the research study is sufficiently powerful to be able to provide conclusive evidence of the relative benefits of the treatments being compared.

References

1   Halpin DMG, Ferenbach C, Bellamy D *et al.* on behalf of the British Thoracic Society COPD Consortium (2002) *What Does the General Public Know About COPD?* Poster presentation at the British Thoracic Society conference, accessed on www.brit-thoracic.org.uk/copd/pdf/posters_prens/Halpin%20abstract.doc

2   Calverley PMA and Walker P (2003) Chronic obstructive pulmonary disease. *Lancet.* **362:** 1053–61.

3   Office for National Statistics (1999) *Mortality Statistics; Cause: England and Wales 1998.* Government Statistical Service, London.

4   Price D and Duerden M (2003) Chronic obstructive pulmonary disease [editorial]. *British Medical Journal.* **326:** 1046–7.

5   Workshop report from the NHLBI/WHO Workshop (updated 2003) *Global Strategy for the Diagnosis, Management and Prevention of COPD: a pocket guide.* Zambon Group at www.goldcopd.com

6   National Institute for Clinical Excellence (2004) *National Clinical Guideline on Management of Chronic Obstructive Pulmonary Disease in Adults in Primary and Secondary Care.* National Institute for Clinical Excellence, London. Slide kit of guidelines downloadable from www.brit-thoracic.org.uk/copd

7   www.brit-thoracic.org.uk/copd/consortium.html

8   The British Thoracic Society (1997) COPD Guidelines Summary. *Thorax.* **52 (suppl. 5):** S1–S32. www.brit-thoracic.org.uk/copd/pdf/COPDSummary.pdf

9   Foord-Kelcey G (ed.) (2003) COPD diagnosis, management and prevention. *Guidelines.* **20:** 83–7. www.eguidelines.co.uk

10   The British Thoracic Society COPD Consortium (2000) *Spirometry in Practice.* Direct Publishing Solutions Ltd, Berks.

11   Munafo M, Drury M, Wakley G *et al.* (2003) *Smoking Cessation Matters in Primary Care.* Radcliffe Medical Press, Oxford.

12   Riemsma RP, Pattenden J, Bridle C *et al.* (2003) Systematic review of the effectiveness of stage based interventions to promote smoking cessation. *British Medical Journal.* **326:** 1175–7.

13 Morgan MDL on behalf of the British Thoracic Society Standards of Care Subcommittee on Pulmonary Rehabilitation (2001) Pulmonary rehabilitation. *Thorax.* **56:** 827–34.

14 Barr RG, Rowe BH and Camargo CA (2003) Methylxanthines for exacerbations of chronic obstructive pulmonary disease: meta-analysis of randomised trials. *British Medical Journal.* **327:** 646–51.

15 Hermiz O, Comino E, Marks G *et al.* (2002) Randomised controlled trial of home based care of patients with chronic obstructive pulmonary disease. *British Medical Journal.* **325:** 938.

16 The BTS COPD Consortium (2003) *Managing Advanced COPD.* BMA Publishing, London. www.brit-thoracic.org.uk

17 The British Thoracic Society and British Lung Foundation (2002) *Pulmonary Rehabilitation Survey.* The British Thoracic Society and British Lung Foundation, London.

18 Godlee F (ed.) (2004) *Clinical Evidence Concise.* BMJ Publishing Group, London. www.clinicalevidence.com

6

Depression

Episodes of 'major' depression are twice as common in women as men. Major depression is strongly associated with adverse life and economic circumstances – such as unemployment, divorce or poor housing. Depression is the most common mental health problem in older people, especially those living in nursing and residential care. 10–15% of older adults aged over 65 years have significant depressive symptoms, although major depression is rare. Women are more likely to be depressed than men. Depressive symptoms are the fourth most important cause of disability worldwide. In the UK:

- about 90% of mental healthcare is delivered solely in primary care[1]
- depression accounts for 10% of all new diagnoses in primary care[2]
- antidepressant drugs account for 7% of UK primary care drug expenditure[2]
- untreated depressed patients use two to three times the annual medical services compared to their non-depressed counterparts[3]
- depression is a stronger predictor of serious cardiac disease during the year following cardiac catheterisation than smoking, severity of coronary artery disease and diminished left ventricular ejection fraction.[4]

It is generally held that GPs fail to diagnose up to half of cases of depression or anxiety. However, longitudinal studies have shown that most patients who did not receive a diagnosis of depression at a single consultation were given a diagnosis at subsequent consultations, or recovered without a GP's diagnosis.[5] GPs seem least likely to miss severe episodes of major depression – much of what is missed is mild and likely to improve spontaneously. Depression or other mental ill-health should not be considered as a stand-alone diagnosis. It often co-exists with physical, emotional and social problems and other psychiatric disorders such as alcohol and drug misuse, anxiety, obsessive–compulsive disorders and eating disorders.[6–9]

One study of frequent attenders to general practice found that depressive symptoms were the major predictor of frequent attendance rather than physical health problems.[10]

Case study 6.1

You recognise Mrs Down as she enters your consulting room. You know that, in the past, she suffered from two episodes of depression requiring treatment with antidepressants. Looking at her records, you see that she took tricyclic antidepressants for three months for both episodes. The last episode was about two years ago. She looks gloomy as she sits down and in response to your usual opening of 'How are you today?' promptly bursts into tears.

What issues you should cover[11–13]

Depression affects the majority of people at some time – so Mrs Down is in good company. Around 60–70% of adults will experience depression or worry of sufficient severity to influence their daily activities at some time in their lives.[11–13] Episodes of depression are short-lived for most people.

Depression is one of the most common reasons for consulting a GP. Up to 50% of people attending general practice may have some depressive symptoms, of whom 5–10% have 'major' depression (*see* Box 6.1). The majority of people with depression are treated and managed in primary care. For a GP with an average list size of 1800 patients, there will be 111 working age adults with depression and/or anxiety warranting treatment and 40 older people with depression.

Symptoms and signs of depression[11]

Symptoms are summarised in Box 6.1. Depression and anxiety often present together. Physical symptoms may be the presenting feature(s) of depression and lead to delayed or missed diagnoses of depression. Several times as many people have one or some depressive symptoms as meet the criteria for major depression.[12]

Box 6.1:   Criteria for 'major' depression[11]

At least five of the symptoms listed below must be present most of the day or nearly every day, during a two week period, of which at least one must be 'depressed mood' or 'diminished interest or pleasure':

- depressed mood
- markedly diminished interest or pleasure in normal activities
- significant weight loss or gain

- insomnia or hypersomnia
- agitated or retarded
- fatigue or loss of energy
- feelings of worthlessness or excessive guilt
- diminished ability to think or concentrate, or indecisiveness
- recurrent thoughts of death or suicidal thoughts or actions.

The presentation of depression in people over 65 years old may be atypical, with low mood being masked. The patient may present with anxiety or memory impairment. The symptoms may be due to dementia, as depression and dementia commonly co-exist.

Depression may be 'bipolar' or 'unipolar'. The term 'bipolar' describes depression that occurs in conjunction with manic episodes. Other depression is termed 'unipolar' – as Box 6.2 describes.

Box 6.2:   Classification of primary depression

Unipolar

- Single depressive episode:
    - mild, moderate or severe
    - with or without somatic syndrome
    - if severe, with or without psychotic symptoms
- Mixed anxiety and depressive disorder
- Recurrent depressive disorder
- Brief recurrent depression
- Seasonal affective disorder
- Dysthymia: depression intermittently for more than two years that does not fulfil criteria for mild or moderate depressive episode.

Bipolar

- Bipolar affective disorder
- Cyclothymia: persistent instability of mood

Course of the illness[12]

About half the people who have major depression experience a further depressive episode in the following 10 years.

- *Mild to moderate depression*: sufferers have depressive symptoms and some functional impairment. Many recover in the short term, and about half have recurrent symptoms.
- *Severe depression*: sufferers have depressive symptoms plus agitation or psychomotor retardation and somatic symptoms.
- *Psychotic depression*: sufferers have hallucinations, delusions or both in addition to their depressive symptoms.

Case study 6.1 continued

Mrs Down fits with the category mild to moderate depression, and you explain how common it is for depression to recur. She tells you that her brother committed suicide about 10 years previously and she confides that she dreads becoming so depressed that she does the same. You ascertain that although she is depressed she is not having suicidal thoughts.

Suicide and self-harm

Suicide rates are higher in people with depression; it has been estimated that 40–50% of all suicides are committed by people with undiagnosed or inadequately treated depressive disorders.[11] Suicides account for just under 1% of all deaths, of which nearly two-thirds occur in depressed people.[14] Box 6.3 describes the plans in the National Service Framework (NSF) for Mental Health, for preventing suicide; the concepts are generalisable throughout the UK.

Box 6.3:   The approach to preventing suicide via the National Service Framework for England[15]

Local health and social care communities should prevent suicides by:

- *Standard one*: promoting mental health for all, working with individuals and communities
- *Standard two*: delivering high quality primary mental healthcare
- *Standard three*: ensuring that anyone with a mental health problem can contact local services via the primary care team, a helpline or an emergency department

- *Standard four*: ensuring that individuals with severe and enduring mental illness have a care plan which meets their specific needs, including access to services round the clock
- *Standard five*: providing safe hospital accommodation for individuals who need it
- *Standard six*: enabling individuals caring for someone with severe mental illness to receive the support that they need to continue to care
- *Standard seven*: in addition to the above:
  - supporting local prison staff in preventing suicides among prisoners
  - ensuring that staff are competent to assess the risk of suicide among individuals at greatest risk
  - developing local systems for suicide to learn lessons and take any necessary action.

Deliberate self-harm involves intentional self-poisoning or injury. It is one of the top five causes of acute medical admissions for both women and men in the UK. Around 50–60% of patients have visited their GP in the month before the episode of their self-harm.[16]

Risk factors for suicide include: unemployment, low income, being single and a history of mental illness necessitating hospital admission. High-risk groups include: the mentally ill, those with a history of parasuicide, alcoholics, prisoners and certain occupational groups such as doctors, pharmacists, farmers and vets. Methods used to commit suicide include overdose (24%), hanging (20%) and car exhaust fumes (20%).[14]

The target for year 2010 in England is to reduce the death rate from suicide and undetermined injury by at least a fifth – saving 4000 lives.[15]

Recommendations for psychiatric referral

Referral to psychiatric services is indicated:

- if there is a risk of suicide
- for psychotic symptoms
- with a history of a bipolar affective disorder
- when the practitioner feels insufficiently experienced to manage a patient's condition
- if two or more attempts to treat the patient's depressive disorder have failed or resulted in only partial response.

Case study 6.1 continued

Mrs Down asks you if she can try something different this time to 'cure' her depression as the last lot of antidepressants do not seem to have worked since her depression is back again. You explain to Mrs Down that she did not complete either of the previous two courses of antidepressants, as she did not return to consult you once she started to feel better and stopped taking her prescribed treatment. You therefore advise her to try a full course of anti-depressant drugs this time, continuing with the treatment for at least four to six months after she starts to feel better, consulting you regularly over that period.

Treatment of depressive disorders

You discuss with Mrs Down that there are two main approaches to treating depression:

1 psychological treatment (counselling or cognitive behavioural therapy)
2 medical treatment with antidepressant drugs.

Psychological treatments may be sufficient for mild forms of depression. For moderate or severe depression, antidepressants alone or in combination with psychological treatments may be appropriate. The evidence for the different approaches in the treatment of depressive disorders that are effective or likely to be beneficial is outlined in Box 6.4.

Box 6.4:   Effective interventions for depression[12,17,18,19]

- *Medication*:
    - tricyclic and heterocyclic antidepressants (in mild, moderate and severe depression)
    - monoamine oxidase inhibitors (in mild, moderate and severe depression)
    - selective serotonin reuptake inhibitors (SSRIs) and related drugs (in mild, moderate and severe depression)
    - St John's Wort (in mild to moderate depression)
    - continuation treatment with antidepressant drugs (reduces risk of re-lapse in mild to moderate depression)
- *Psychotherapy*:
    - cognitive therapy (in mild to moderate depression)
    - interpersonal therapy (in mild to moderate depression)
    - problem-solving therapy (in mild to moderate depression)
- *Combined medication and psychotherapy* (in mild, moderate and severe depression)

- *Electroconvulsive therapy* (in severe depression)
- *Other approaches*:
  - care pathways (in mild to moderate depression)

There is a vast array of antidepressants available and while a great deal of evidence exists for the effectiveness of SSRIs and tricyclic antidepressants, there is less evidence for the effectiveness of other neurotransmitter drugs. These others include drugs chemically related to, but different from, the tricyclic antidepressants such as trazodone and a range of other chemically unrelated antidepressants including mirtazapine. Other drugs used either alone or in combination with antidepressant drugs include lithium salts and the antipsychotics, although use of these drugs is usually reserved for people with severe, psychotic or chronic depression.[14]

The choice of antidepressant will be based on the individual person's requirements, including the presence of co-existing disease, current therapy, suicide risk and previous response to antidepressant medication. For instance, tricyclic drugs should be prescribed with special caution in people with epilepsy (as they lower the convulsive threshold) or with cardiac disease (as occasionally arrhythmias and heart block may occur).

Lithium should only be prescribed by a specialist. The potential risks and benefits should be carefully weighed and the need for continued therapy regularly re-assessed. The primary care team should monitor the dose carefully because of the narrow therapeutic range and potential toxicity. The primary care team should monitor lithium levels every three months. The practice protocol for the management of lithium should be set up to recall patients every three months, so that blood tests can be arranged 12 hours postdose. Serum creatinine and thyroid stimulating hormone (TSH) should be checked every 6–12 months, as hypothyroidism and abnormal renal function are relatively common side-effects. Other problems that can arise include blurred vision, vomiting, dysarthria, ataxia, coarse tremor, reduced sex drive, drowsiness, confusion, seizures, coma and hypotension. Patients should be warned not to stop lithium abruptly, to avoid a rebound psychosis.

Figure 6.1 describes current guidelines for managing depression in primary care, updated by the British Association of Psychopharmacology (BAP).[17] These guidelines emphasise the importance of choosing an antidepressant drug that best suits the individual patient. There are several national clinical practice guidelines for depressive disorders. A review of such guidelines found 15, of which the BAP guidelines are one.[20]

SSRIs or tricyclic antidepressants are more effective than placebo in the treatment of major and minor depressive disorders.[12] Antidepressants are more effective than placebo in the treatment of chronic mild depressive disorders.[12,14]

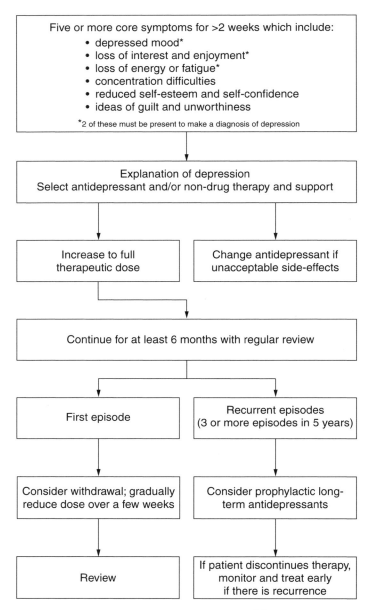

Figure 6.1:   Current management guidance for depression[17]

When SSRIs are compared with tricyclic antidepressants in people with all grades of depression there is no clinically significant difference in effectiveness.[12,21] Research comparing side-effects of SSRIs and tricyclics found that tricyclic antidepressants were associated with higher rates of adverse effects, but the difference was small.[12] Abrupt withdrawal of SSRIs is associated with symptoms such as dizziness, nausea, paraesthesia, headache and vertigo.[12]

Monoamine oxidase inhibitors (MAOIs) are occasionally used as second-line drugs and must be used with caution because of the potential serious adverse effect of a hypertensive crisis occurring without dietary limitation. Compared with tricyclic drugs, MAOIs are less effective in treating severe depressive disorders, but more effective in treating atypical depressive disorders, characterised by increased sleep, increased appetite, mood reactivity, and rejection sensitivity.[12]

Antidepressant medication is highly effective when used properly, but depression is often inadequately treated and depressed patients may receive either no medication or sub-therapeutic doses of medication – as in Mrs Down's case.[22]

The array of clinical practice guidelines that exist for depression focus mainly on major depression, rather than the mild to moderate depression that is commonly seen in primary care. This does limit their applicability and relevance to those working in primary care and the types of patients being treated in primary as opposed to secondary care.

Case study 6.1 continued

You work hard to inform Mrs Down about the rationale for treating depression with medication, and the benefits and risks of treatments, to gain her concordance. You discuss the dose and different types of antidepressant drugs and the possibility of continuing medication to prevent a future return of her depression. After your discussion Mrs Down feels that she could make an informed choice and elects to try an SSRI, which might have fewer side-effects than the tricyclic drug she had taken before, and you agree to meet monthly. You discuss starting cognitive therapy as well as taking the medication, to help to prevent relapse.

Prescribing tips

From compliance to concordance

Research has shown that up to 8% of prescriptions for antidepressants are never dispensed.[23] Many drugs that are dispensed are not consumed. At least 25–50% of patients on antidepressant medication take irregular or insufficient doses. So you should find ways to encourage patients to adhere to the drugs prescribed, by giving them better information so that they can take part in the decision to take antidepressants and be more likely to 'own' that agreement. Understanding the differences between compliance and concordance may help doctors and nurses to structure a negotiated agreement rather than issue instructions to the patient.

In the past, the term 'non-compliance' was used to highlight the situation when many patients were unable or unwilling to take their medication as prescribed. However, the term 'non-compliance' portrays the unequal partnership between patients and health professionals. Implicit in the term 'compliance' is the idea that patients take orders from health professionals.

Concordance describes a two-way communication that recognises that the health beliefs of the patient, although different from those of doctor, nurse or pharmacist, are no less valuable or important in deciding the best approach to the treatment of the individual. Concordance is a therapeutic partnership reached between the patient and the healthcare professional following negotiation, that respects the beliefs and wishes of the patient even if that means that he/she decides not to take their medicine or to alter their treatment in some way.[23,24]

Keep dosing schedules as simple as possible to aid concordance. Patients should be counselled that it usually takes at least two weeks for them to notice any benefit from antidepressants.[19]

Dose

SSRI drugs can be started at the recommended maintenance dose except in the elderly where it is wise to start with half the normal adult dose and titrate upwards as necessary to gain clinical improvement. As most side-effects vary with dose, gradually increase the dose until side-effects appear and then slowly decrease the dose until they disappear or are tolerable.[18,19]

MAOIs should not be prescribed within six weeks of discontinuing fluoxetine because of its long half-life, within two weeks of paroxetine, mirtazapine and sertraline, or within one week of citalopram, fluvoxamine and venlafaxine.

Dependence and withdrawal

Reassure patients that antidepressants are not addictive. Once an antidepressant has been taken for more than a few weeks, there should be at least a planned four-week tapering off period when they are discontinued to avoid any reaction. The abrupt withdrawal of SSRIs such as paroxetine and fluvoxamine, which have a short half-life, can lead to a 'discontinuation syndrome' in up to one in five patients. This is characterised by transient flu-like symptoms including dizziness, nausea, paraesthesia, headache, tremor, palpitations, vertigo and anxiety.[12] Withdrawal reactions have been reported more frequently for paroxetine than for sertraline and fluoxetine.[12]

Continuation and maintenance treatment

Continuing treatment with antidepressant drugs for 4–6 months after recovery (in mild or moderate depression) reduces the risk of relapse by almost half; for the elderly this period should be extended to 12 months.[12]

Maintain long-term treatment for recurrent depressive disorder in order to prevent the recurrence of further depressive episodes. Several trials have found that maintenance treatment reduces the relapse rate in recurrent depressive disorder compared with placebo.[12]

Consider maintenance or prophylactic treatment with antidepressant drugs for people who have had three or more recent episodes of significant depression or more than five episodes all together.

Other non-prescribed medication treatments

Electroconvulsive therapy

Electroconvulsive therapy (ECT) is effective in treating patients with acute severe depressive disorder.[12] ECT is a short-term treatment that may be useful when a rapid response is required. People often complain of memory impairment following ECT. ECT should be reserved for those who cannot tolerate drugs or who have not responded to other treatment, where a rapid response is required in severe depression considered to be life-threatening or in catatonia, a prolonged or severe manic episode.[25]

Specific psychological treatments

Interpersonal psychotherapy, problem-solving therapy and non-directive counselling have been found to be as effective as drugs in treating mild to moderate depression in people of all ages.[12]

Cognitive behavioural therapy

This is a 'talking' therapy used for people suffering from depression, anxiety and eating disorders.[12] In cognitive behavioural therapy (CBT), links are made between the person's feelings and patterns of thinking that underpin their distress. The patient is encouraged to take an active part in examining the evidence for and against distressing beliefs, challenging the habitual patterns of thinking about the belief and using reasoning and personal experience to develop rational and acceptable alternatives. Therapy may typically be carried out as 20 sessions over 12 to 16 weeks with some occasional follow-up booster sessions.[12] It is provided by clinical psychologists, psychiatrists or community psychiatric nurses.

Cognitive therapy focuses on changing the dysfunctional beliefs and negative automatic thoughts that characterise depressive disorders. One review of published research demonstrated that cognitive therapy may be more effective than drug treatment in people with mild to moderate depression.[12]

Interpersonal psychotherapy

Interpersonal therapy (IPT) is a brief, standardised treatment for depression, which usually consists of 12–16 weekly sessions.[12] IPT is primarily used for people with unipolar non-psychotic depressive disorders. The therapeutic techniques employed focus on improving the patient's interpersonal functioning within current relationships and identifying the problems associated with the onset of the depressive episode in order to prevent relapse. Patients are initially educated about the nature of depression and reassured that their various symptoms are part of their depression. The depressive symptoms are addressed in a similar fashion to the behavioural techniques used in cognitive behavioural therapy. The therapist then moves on to address the interpersonal issues relevant for that individual. The main problem areas are then defined and become the focus of therapy.[18]

Problem solving

Problem solving is briefer and simpler than cognitive therapy and so may be feasible within a primary care setting.[12] It consists of three stages:

1 identifying the main problems for the patient
2 generating solutions
3 trying out the solutions.

Non-directive counselling

This was developed by Rogers in 1961 and aims to help people to express feelings and to clarify thoughts and difficulties.[26] The therapist does not give direct advice, but suggests alternative understandings and encourages people to solve their own problems.

St John's Wort (hypericum perforatum)

St John's Wort is more effective than placebo in the treatment of mild to moderate depressive disorders and is as effective as prescription antidepressant drugs. However, this evidence must be interpreted with caution as the research upon which this report is based was not undertaken on fully representative groups of people using standardised preparations, and doses of antidepressants varied.[12,27]

Acupuncture

Acupuncture may relieve depressive symptoms. Three Chinese trials indicated that acupuncture was as effective as tricyclic antidepressant drugs in relieving depression.[27]

Exercise

There is limited evidence that exercise, alone or combined with other treatments, is beneficial in mild to moderate depression.[12]

Screening for depression

None of the definitions and scores that can categorise depression are used routinely in primary care.[28] Research suggests that most depression that GPs treat is below, or just reaches, the minimum diagnostic criteria for major depression (*see* Box 6.1). GPs appear to see their patients in terms of 'fluctuating mood disturbances occurring in response to life situations, often against the background of chronic difficulties, physical illness, insecure relationships and deprivation'.[28]

Validated screening questionnaires cannot be recommended for systematic screening. They tend to be used in research on depression in primary care but there is no convincing evidence that identifying cases via validated questionnaires, such as the Beck Depression Inventory or the Geriatric Depression Scale, improves clinical outcomes.[29,30] The presence of depression should be confirmed by clinical assessment of the state of the person's mental health.

Quality indicators in mental health[31]

Depression is a chronic disease that requires quality management as an essential service of general practice. This includes relevant health promotion, treatment and referral. Mental health is one of the 10 domains of chronic disease management specified within the GMS contract. Table 6.1 lists the quality indicators relevant to mental health and associated points. People with 'severe long-term mental health problems' are described in the NSF as 'patients who are managed by the care plan approach'.[15] These may include patients:

- suffering from severe or recurrent depression
- suffering from bipolar depression
- with a history of psychosis
- with drug and/or alcohol addiction.

It is not explicit whether all PCOs will include severe and enduring depression within the umbrella of 'severe long-term mental health problems' or will assume the term mainly applies to schizophrenia.

Table 6.1:   Quality indicators in mental health

Indicator		Points	Maximum threshold (%)
MH1	The practice can produce a register of people with severe long-term mental health problems who require and have agreed to regular follow-up.	7	
MH2	The percentage of patients with severe long-term mental health problems with a review recorded in the preceding 15 months. This review includes a check on the accuracy of prescribed medication, a review of physical health and a review of co-ordination arrangements with secondary care.	23	90
MH3	The percentage of patients on lithium therapy with a record of lithium levels checked within the previous 6 months.	3	90
MH4	The percentage of patients on lithium therapy with a record of serum creatinine and TSH in the preceding 15 months.	3	90
MH5	The percentage of patients on lithium therapy with a record of lithium levels in the therapeutic range within the previous 6 months.	5	70

All minimum thresholds are 25%

Practices may contract to provide enhanced services covering the specialised care of depression. These practices should be able to:

- produce and maintain an up-to-date register of depressed patients
- apply a multidisciplinary approach
- use cognitive behavioural therapy
- use screening procedures
- undertake appropriate training
- maintain personal health plans
- make referrals and inquiries as clinically indicated
- perform an annual review
- receive feedback from patients and their families using an appropriate questionnaire.

Collecting data to demonstrate your learning, competence, performance and standards of service delivery

Example cycle of evidence 6.1

- Focus: clinical care
- Other relevant foci: relationships with patients; working with colleagues

Stages of the evidence cycle

Stage 1 — Select targets

Stage 2 — Set standards

Stage 3A/B — Identify needs

Stage 4 — Learning/action plan

Stage 5 — Document it all

Case study 6.2

Ms Sadd comes to see you, cuddling her nine-month-old baby to her in a sling. She sits down and bursts into tears. She is finding it increasingly difficult to get through her work in the local tourist information service and look after her son, as she is so tired. Her partner works away from home so she feels like a single parent, always being the one to take and collect her son from nursery and look after him when he's sick. Her work is suffering and she was disciplined last week for losing her temper with customers. She asks for tablets to help her to sleep better so that she can cope with work and as a mum.

This is just an example. Keep your task simple. You could choose three or four cycles of evidence to demonstrate your competence each year.

Stage 1: Select your aspirations for good practice

The excellent GP:

- takes time to elicit all relevant details of a patient's history
- explains the diagnosis to a patient so that they can make an informed choice about treatment and management options.

Stage 2: Set the standards for your outcomes

Outcomes might include:

- the way learning is applied
- a learnt skill
- a protocol
- a strategy that is implemented
- meeting recommended standards.

- Agree a practice protocol with the health visitors and GP colleagues for managing women with postnatal depression.
- Map out the local support services available to women with postnatal depression.

Stage 3A: Identify your learning needs

- Self-assess whether you are up to date with treatment of postnatal depression.
- Carry out a significant event audit of a patient who was diagnosed with postnatal depression by a GP colleague when the baby was one year old. You had seen the patient for back pain and you realise looking back that the patient had postnatal depression for many months.

Stage 3B: Identify your service needs

> Any of the needs assessment exercises in 3A may also reveal service needs.

- Discuss the findings of the significant event audit in 3A (second point) as a team at an educational meeting in the practice. Check whether all members of the team are aware of services available to women with postnatal depression, e.g. benefit payments, psychological therapies, Sure Start, Home Start, childcare centres etc.
- Audit the extent to which women who have been treated for postnatal depression in the previous 12 months have been followed up by the team or by an individual person.

Stage 4: Make and carry out a learning and action plan

- Arrange a tutorial with a health visitor with a special interest in postnatal depression, to include the use of a screening questionnaire.
- Run an educational session in the practice where you present best practice guidance for managing postnatal depression after reading up on the topic and the tutorial with the health visitor. You present a draft protocol for managing postnatal depression, which is discussed and agreed by those present. The session culminates by the team pooling their knowledge to map out the support services available for women with postnatal depression.

Stage 5: Document your learning, competence, performance and standards of service delivery

- Draw a flow diagram of the services available to women with postnatal depression.
- Include the updated and agreed practice protocol for managing postnatal depression.

- Audit the extent of the follow-up for patients with postnatal depression, including the proportion on medication who continue on medication for at least six months. Include any necessary action plan.
- Record the discussions and conclusions from the significant event audit of the delay in recognition of postnatal depression and the reasons for the delayed diagnosis.

Case study 6.2 continued

Ms Sadd accepts your diagnosis of depression. She considers the options of no treatment, taking antidepressant tablets and/or seeing a community psychiatric nurse for counselling, and opts for antidepressant medication. She prefers to continue at work and not take sickness leave. The health visitor goes round to see Ms Sadd at home on her day off work and their discussion and her advice help Ms Sadd to understand her feelings and make a practical plan with her partner to relieve some of the pressure she is under from working almost full-time and acting as a single parent.

Example cycle of evidence 6.2

- Focus: good medical practice
- Other relevant foci: confidentiality; consent

Stages of the evidence cycle

Stage 1
Select targets

Stage 2
Set standards

Stage 5
Document it all

Stage 3A/B
Identify needs

Stage 4
Learning/action plan

Case study 6.3

Jack comes to see you in surgery in place of his mother, Mrs Lowe. You have her name on the appointment slot and her notes on your computer screen. He explains that he lives 10 miles from his mother, and sees her about once a month. She rarely goes out and he made the appointment for her because he was worried that she is not eating and is losing weight and often smells as if she's been drinking sherry. She used to be house proud but her house is now untidy and she just does not seem to care about the mess. Since her husband died two years ago, she's become more and more of a recluse. He doesn't feel he can do any more and Mrs Lowe tearfully refused to come with him to see you, the GP – she just asked to be left alone.

> This is just an example. Keep your task simple. You could choose three or four cycles of evidence to demonstrate your competence each year.

Stage 1: Select your aspirations for good practice

The excellent GP:

- is sure about the limits of confidentiality when talking to a person about another patient without their explicit permission
- is confident about diagnosing mental illness
- provides proactive care to patients suffering from depression.

Stage 2: Set the standards for your outcomes

Outcomes might include:

- the way learning is applied
- a learnt skill
- a protocol
- a strategy that is implemented
- meeting recommended standards.

- Devise a specific action plan for seeking out patients who are reported to have health problems about which they refuse to consult.

- An audit shows that you are alert to potential contraindications to the prescribing of antidepressants to people who are elderly or consuming excessive alcohol.

Stage 3A: Identify your learning needs

- Keep a reflective diary noting down your suspicions of co-existing mental ill-health as patients present with physical symptoms. Compare your reflections with what is revealed at successive consultations with you or your colleagues.
- Invite feedback from colleagues about whether your care of elderly patients is appropriate, e.g. from district nurses, other GPs, health visitors, receptionists.
- Review how you would or could diagnose depression with the community psychiatric nurse. Invite her to comment on gaps in your knowledge.

Stage 3B: Identify your service needs

Any of the needs assessment exercises in 3A may also reveal service needs.

- Review the consultation pattern of patients of all age groups both in surgery and from home visits. Compare the consultation rates of elderly people with younger age groups. Identify any barriers contributing to the differences in consultation rates.
- Invite feedback from individual older people and people suffering from mental illness. You could include prompts about the ease of access to the surgery, e.g. physical access, times of surgery sessions, availability of particular GPs and nurses, transport from across the geographical area etc.
- Carry out a significant event audit arising from a breach of confidentiality relating to one of the practice team giving out patient-specific information to a relative without explicit consent from the patient concerned.

Stage 4: Make and carry out a learning and action plan

- Continue the discussion of the gaps with the community psychiatric nurse with a tutorial on best practice in managing depression, especially alternative approaches to medication.
- Discuss the feedback from older patients and those with mental illness with patients on your practice patient panel, to determine if they agree with the findings, and if so, debate possible improvements.
- Read up on care pathways for mild to moderate depression. Convene a working group of local primary care clinicians and psychiatrists to discuss composing a care pathway with backing from the PCO.

- Phone the medical director of the PCO to discuss problems and issues with confidentiality of patient information where it is difficult to assess the fitness or competence of patients to make decisions about their care (e.g. those with signs of senility, those inebriated, children).

Stage 5: Document your learning, competence, performance and standards of service delivery

- Keep a copy of your draft care pathway.
- Include a copy of the guidance notes for the practice team on handling patient confidentiality where there are complicating issues (*see* Stage 4, point 4, above).
- Include copies of the feedback from patients, and the conclusions and action planned or undertaken to make changes.
- Audit the trends in consultation rates from various population groups such as those with mental health problems.
- Extract anonymised comments from your reflective diary and your planned developments.

Case study 6.3 continued

You explain that you are not able to discuss an able patient with anyone else, including a close relative, without their permission, but you are willing to listen to Jack's concerns about Mrs Lowe and to take what action you consider appropriate. You realise that Mrs Lowe may be at risk from her seeming depression and alcohol misuse and ask the health visitor to visit her at home to undertake an over-75 year old check. The health visitor knows Mrs Lowe already and is able to chat with her about her loneliness, isolation and depression. She brings Mrs Lowe along to surgery to consult you about her depression and arranges for social services to review her social care and needs.

Example cycle of evidence 6.3

- Focus: working with colleagues
- Other relevant focus: health and safety

Stages of the evidence cycle
Stage 1
Select targets

Stage 2
Set standards

Stage 5
Document it all

Stage 3A/B
Identify needs

Stage 4
Learning/action plan

Case study 6.4

Mrs Burden is qualified as a supplementary prescriber in her nurse practitioner role in your practice. Unfortunately she is going through a bad patch at present at home – her mother has a terminal illness, one of her children has been suspended from school and she is recently divorced. She puts a brave face on at work and none of the staff realise that she is depressed. They know that she is forgetful, is rude to patients, makes mistakes in the doses of drugs she is prescribing and takes much longer to do jobs than she used to. The practice manager talks about Mrs Burden's manner at work with you as the GP partner who leads on staff matters, and you both realise that all your concerns relate to the last year – before that Mrs Burden had a different approach to work and you were all pleased with the standards of her work. You offer to chat with her to find out if there's anything going on to account for her changed attitude to work.

This is just an example. Keep your task simple. You could choose three or four cycles of evidence to demonstrate your competence each year.

Stage 1: Select your aspirations for good practice

The excellent GP:

- is interested in and concerned about the health and wellbeing of colleagues at work
- recognises when ill-health factors affect a colleague's work and takes appropriate action.

Stage 2: Set the standards for your outcomes

Outcomes might include:

- the way learning is applied
- a learnt skill
- a protocol
- a strategy that is implemented
- meeting recommended standards.

- The practice policy on health and wellbeing is copied to all practice team members. It describes primary care team members' responsibilities and what action to take when patient safety is at risk.

Stage 3A: Identify your learning needs

- Recall if there has been any similar incident in the past when you feared that a member of staff was under-performing in a way that put patient safety at risk. Identify what action you or others took. Consider if the action was appropriate, could have been improved or a more prompt response made.
- Discuss the nature of an employer's responsibility for under-performing staff with the practice manager, who worked previously as a manager in industry in charge of many staff.

Stage 3B: Identify your service needs

> Any of the needs assessment exercises in 3A may also reveal service needs.

- Find out what occupational health services exist for primary care staff in your locality, and if staff know how to access occupational health services or refer others to them.
- Assess the content and application of your practice's health and safety policy, especially the items that relate to staff health. How easy was it to find your policy? When was it last reviewed or amended? Compare the content against a best practice checklist, for example, look at *Occupational Health Matters in General Practice*.[32]

Stage 4: Make and carry out a learning and action plan

- Discuss the updated practice health and safety policy with a local GP with an occupational health post at a local factory. Make final revisions and detailed additions about the health and wellbeing of staff.
- Book dedicated time for discussion with the practice manager about employers' responsibilities in respect of the ill-health of staff and their rehabilitation.
- Read up about patient safety in the National Patient Safety Agency's literature.[33]

Stage 5: Document your learning, competence, performance and standards of service delivery

- Include the revised practice policy for health and safety and wellbeing of staff.
- Make a poster of the practice 'charter' about patient safety for the wall of the staff room.
- Include factual and contemporaneous notes about staff giving concern (anonymised for your portfolio), the discussions, and the agreed action by the employer (you or the practice manager) and the staff member with follow-up records.

Case study 6.4 continued

Soon after you start to discuss the mistakes that Mrs Burden has made with prescribing, it becomes obvious to you that she has health problems that may be linked to her performance at work. You therefore halt the discussion and advise Mrs Burden to consult her own GP. She makes an appointment the next day and experienced a great relief at being able to unburden herself and not keep up her 'front'. Her GP signed her off sick for two weeks and offered her treatment for her depression. Two months later, she returns to work after receiving the okay from the trust's occupational health department, a much happier person and a more effective nurse.

References

1   Goldberg DP and Huxley P (1980) *Mental Illness in the Community: the pathways to psychiatric care.* Tavistock Publications, London.

2   Peveler R, George C, Kinmouth A *et al.* (1999) Effect of anti-depressant drug counselling and information leaflets on adherence to drug treatment in primary care: randomised controlled trial. *British Medical Journal.* **319:** 612–15.

3   Simon G, von Korff M and Barlow W (1995) Health care costs of primary care patients with recognised depression. *Archives of General Psychiatry.* **52:** 850–6.

4   Carney RM, Rich MW, Freedland KE *et al.* (1988) Major depressive disorder predicts cardiac events in patients with coronary artery disease. *Psychosomatic Medicine.* **50:** 627–33.

5   Kessler D, Bennewith O, Lewis G *et al.* (2002) Detection of depression and anxiety in primary care: follow up study. *British Medical Journal.* **325:** 1016–17.

6   Barrett J, Oxman T and Gerber P (1988) The prevalence of psychiatric disorders in primary care practice. *Archives of General Practice.* **45:** 1100–6.

7   Bridges KW and Goldberg DP (1985) Somatic presentation of DSM III psychiatric disorders in primary care. *Journal of Psychosomatic Research.* **29:** 563–9.

8   Chambers R, Boath E and Wakley G (2001) *Mental Health Matters in Primary Care.* Radcliffe Medical Press, Oxford.

9   Katon W, von Korff M, Lin E *et al.* (1992) A randomised trial of psychiatric consultation with distressed high utilisers. *General Hospital Psychiatry.* **14:** 86–98.

10 Dowrick C, Bellon J and Gomez M (2000) GP frequent attendance in Liverpool and Granada: the impact of depressive symptoms. *British Journal of General Practice.* **50:** 361–5.

11 Freemantle N, Long A, Mason J *et al.* (1993) The treatment of depression in primary care. *Effective Health Care Bulletin.* **5**, University of Leeds, Leeds.

12 Godlee F (ed.) (2004) *Clinical Evidence.* Issue 11. BMJ Publishing Group, London.

13 Collier J (2000) The management of postnatal depression. *Drug and Therapeutics Bulletin.* **38(5):** 33–7.

14 National Collaborating Centre for Mental Health (2003) *Depression: the management of depression in primary and secondary care.* Draft for second consultation.

National Clinical Practice Guideline Development Group for the National Institute for Clinical Excellence, London.

15 National Health Service Executive (2000) *National Service Framework for Mental Health*. Department of Health, London.

16 House A, Owens D and Patchett L (1998) Deliberate self-harm. *Effective Health Care Bulletin*. **4(6)**, University of York, York.

17 Anderson IM, Nutt DJ and Deakin JFW (2000) Evidence based guidelines for treating depressive disorders with antidepressants: a revision of the 1983 British Association for Psychopharmacology guidelines. *Journal of Psychopharmacology*. **14:** 3–20, in: G Foord-Kelcey (ed.) *Guidelines in Practice*. **21:** 151–4.

18 Joint Formulary Committee (2004) *British National Formulary*. BNF 47. British Medical Association and Royal Pharmaceutical Society of Great Britain, London.

19 Wilkinson G, Moore B and Moore P (2000) *Treating People with Depression*. Radcliffe Medical Press, Oxford.

20 Cornwall P and Scott J (2000) Which clinical practice guidelines for depression? An overview for busy practitioners. *British Journal of General Practice*. **50:** 908–11.

21 MacGillivray S, Arroll B, Hatcher S *et al.* (2003) Efficacy and tolerability of selective serotonin reuptake inhibitors compared with tricyclic antidepressants in depression treated in primary care: systematic review and meta-analysis. *British Medical Journal*. **326:** 1014–17.

22 Lepine JP, Gastpar M, Mendlewicz J *et al.* (1997) Depression in the community: the first pan-European study DEPRES (Depression Research in European Society). *International Clinical Psychopharmacology*. **12(1):** 19–29.

23 Johnston D (1981) Depression: treatment compliance in general practice. *Acta Psychiatrica Scandinavica*. **Suppl. 63:** 447–53.

24 Marinker M (ed.) (1997) *From Compliance to Concordance: achieving shared goals in medicine taking*. Royal Pharmaceutical Society; Merck, Sharp, and Dohme, London.

25 National Institute for Clinical Excellence (2003) Guidance on the use of electroconvulsive therapy. *Technology Appraisal*. **59**, National Institute for Clinical Excellence, London.

26 Rogers CR (1961) *On Becoming a Person*. Houghton Mifflin, Boston.

27 Ernst E (ed.) (2001) *Complementary and Alternative Medicine – a desktop reference*. Harcourt Health Sciences, London.

28 Collier J (ed.) (2003) Mild depression in general practice: time for a rethink? *Drugs and Therapeutics Bulletin*. **41(8):** 60–4.

29 Armstrong E (1997) *Primary Mental Health Care Toolkit*. Royal College of General Practitioners Unit for Mental Health Education in Primary Care, London.

30 NHS Centre for Reviews and Dissemination (2002) Improving the recognition and management of depression in primary care. *Effective Health Care Bulletin*. **7**, University of York, York.

31   General Practitioners Committee/The NHS Confederation (2003) *New GMS Contract. Investing in general practice.* General Practitioners Committee/NHS Confederation, London.

32   Chambers R, Moore S, Parker G and Slovak A (2001) *Occupational Health Matters in General Practice.* Radcliffe Medical Press, Oxford.

33   www.npsa.nhs.uk

7

Dementia

Prevalence of dementia

The prevalence of dementia is difficult to establish. In a Canadian study, the rates varied from 3.1% to 29% of the population studied, depending of which of six systems of diagnosis were used.[1] Pooled data from many studies give the prevalence as shown in Table 7.1.

Table 7.1: Prevalence of dementia in the population in Canada

Age group (years)	Prevalence rate in 100 people
65–69	1.4
70–74	2.8
75–79	5.6
80–84	11.1
85+	23.6

That is, about one in every five people over the age of 80 years suffers from dementia. Most studies show no sex difference in prevalence although some show a slightly higher rate of Alzheimer's disease in women. Regional differences appear in many studies but because of the difficulties of precise classification they give a confusing picture. It is suggested that dementia may be less common in rural than in urban areas, and some types of dementia may be more common in some countries.

Case study 7.1

When you call Mr Grey to the consultation room, you are surprised to see Mrs Grey come in alone. She tells you that she has been increasingly concerned about her husband's mental state. Since he backed the car into the side of the garage, she has been trying to persuade him to stop driving. She has been asking her daughter to pick them up to go shopping, but this involves both her and her daughter in collusion over the reason, or Mr Grey loses his temper and starts shouting. Then last week, a light bulb went in the hall and Mr Grey, who used to do lots of his own repairs around the house, did not seem to know how to change it. When she tried to tell him to leave it, he became quite aggressive and threw the screwdriver he was holding at her. Later he could not understand why she had been crying and said she was exaggerating, the screwdriver must have slipped out of his hand. He has stopped going out every morning to fetch the paper and then making a cup of tea for them both. She gets quite emotional as she tells you how she misses him reading bits of the paper out to her while they drink their tea, although it always used to annoy her!

What issues you should cover

Take Mrs Grey's concerns seriously, even if you think there may be a possibility of marital discord and exaggeration. It helps to have an account from a relative or other informant if you suspect dementia. As dementia progresses, the patient's own awareness and ability to give a clear history diminishes.

Types of dementia

Many people, including some health professionals, lump all mental decline into a broad category of 'dementia' and look no further. It is important to be as precise as possible, both to identify any reversible causes and to make plans for the future.

Dementia can be divided into two main categories. Those conditions where the dementia is reversible include dehydration, vitamin B deficiency due to poor nutrition or secondary to alcohol abuse, hypothyroidism and head injury. Delirium in acute illness, after surgery, or associated with sleep deprivation can be confused with dementia but tends to be of shorter duration and relieved by correction of the precipitating event. Severe depression can sometimes mimic dementia.

Irreversible or progressive conditions include those described in Box 7.1.

Box 7.1:   Irreversible or progressive forms of dementia

* *Alzheimer's disease* (AD): the causes of the brain damage of AD are not yet clear but it is known that abnormal amyloid is laid down in the central nervous system. Most people with rare early onset AD have genetic mutations and it is more common in people with Down's syndrome. Symptoms of AD begin slowly with memory problems and become steadily worse. Over time, the brain damage in AD leads to serious problems in thinking, judgement, and ability to carry out daily activities. Speech and personality are also affected. Impairment of cognitive function is commonly accompanied, and occasionally preceded, by deterioration in emotional control, social behaviour or motivation.[2,3]

- *Lewy body dementia* (LBD): this type of dementia is the possibly second most common cause of dementia in older adults. Lewy bodies are abnormal structures found in certain areas of the brain. This type of dementia can be difficult to diagnose. LBD is characterised by distinct cognitive impairment with fluctuating confusion, disturbance of consciousness, visual hallucinations, delusion, falls and significant parkinsonism. The symptoms tend to come and go, and relatives or professionals may think the individual is pretending to be confused. The condition may be confused with Parkinson's disease because of the symptoms and signs of lack of expression and sensitivity to neuroleptic medication.
- *Multi-infarct or vascular dementia* (MID): in MID, small strokes occur, and blood clots in the blood vessels in the brain cause the death of brain tissue. Symptoms that begin suddenly may be a sign of this kind of dementia. Patients usually have other signs of cardiovascular disease.

The most common form is Alzheimer's disease with about 50–55% of sufferers receiving this diagnosis.[1] About 15–20% have Lewy body or vascular dementia.

There remain around 10% of people with dementia arising from other conditions – about 5% for fronto-temporal dementia including Pick's disease, and another 5% for other dementias including acquired immune deficiency syndrome (AIDS).

- Pick's disease affects the front of the brain, leading to loss of judgement and loss of inhibitions.
- Dementia occurs in the majority of cases of Huntington's disease. This is a hereditary brain disorder causing the loss of cells in the basal ganglia. This cell damage affects cognitive ability (thinking, judgement, memory), movement and emotional control. The symptoms appear gradually, usually in midlife, between the ages of 30 and 50 years.
- Some people with AIDS develop dementia in the later stages of the illness. The AIDS virus itself may attack certain brain cells, and people with AIDS may develop viral infections of the brain because of their weakened immune system.
- The symptoms of Creutzfeldt-Jakob disease (CJD) are similar to those of Alzheimer's disease. An electroencephalogram (EEG) and analysis of the cerebrospinal fluid distinguishes the two conditions.

Clinical priorities

You could invite Mr Grey for a 'well-man' check to assess his physical and mental state. In the early stages of dementia, people may deny that anything is wrong, but sometimes are glad of an opportunity to discuss their fears. In the later stages, people are usually unaware that they have any disability.

Discuss with Mrs Grey whether she feels able to talk to her husband about her concerns about his health. If she can put it in general terms, she may be able to encourage him to attend. However, if Mr Grey has delusions and/or hallucinations, he may have paranoid ideas and be more difficult to help. A history of impairment of function is more likely to imply dementia than just loss of memory.

Identifying and diagnosing dementia[4,5]

It is important not to assume that cognitive impairment equals dementia. A small proportion of people with dementia have an underlying abnormality, such as a brain tumour, that when treated improves cognitive function. Sometimes depression and dementia are confused, particularly in people who become withdrawn and inactive. Depression is common in the early stages of dementia and mental function may improve with treatment of the depression.

Take a history from both the patient and someone who has known the patient for some time. You have the opportunity to hear Mrs Grey's account without Mr Grey being present. This can be important if the patient has delusions, paranoia, denial or is unaware of his dysfunction.

Common causes of cognitive worsening in elderly people are:[6]

- urinary tract, chest, skin or ear infections
- onset or exacerbation of cardiac failure
- drugs, especially prescribed psychiatric or antiparkinsonian drugs and alcohol
- cerebrovascular ischaemia or hypoxia.

Alcohol excess is common in elderly people, especially when they are lonely or lacking in purpose, and other drug use should be considered in some cultures and environments.

Less common causes include:

- severe depression mimicking dementia
- severe anaemia, vitamin B_{12} or folate deficiency
- hypothyroidism
- slow growing cerebral tumour

- renal failure
- communicating hydrocephalus.

Investigations may include:

- full blood count
- erythrocyte sedimentation rate
- urea and electrolytes
- liver function tests (including gamma-glutamyl transferase)
- vitamin B_{12} and folate, if the mean corpuscular volume is raised
- thyroid function test
- midstream urine
- vision and hearing (may contribute to apparent cognitive impairment)
- ECG
- chest X-ray where indicated to exclude pneumonia or possible chest disease
- CT scan: if symptoms are atypical, there is a recent head injury, clinical suspicion of an underlying tumour, new onset of fits, unexplained focal neurological signs or if antidementia drugs are being considered.

Mental state screening instruments

Tests that are widely used to assess cognitive impairment are the mini-mental state examination (MMSE)[4] or the abbreviated mental-test score version,[7] and the six-item cognitive impairment test (6CIT).[8,9] A clock drawing test is becoming increasingly popular and is usually used with the MMSE.[10] Drawing a clock face can reveal deficits in parietal lobe function.

The MMSE consists of 30 questions covering four sections which include: orientation to day, spelling WORLD backwards, recalling three words, and writing a sentence.[4] Take all other factors into consideration when interpreting the result, such as a person's background, culture, education and social class, and information from their carers about how they are functioning. Although the MMSE has its limitations, it represents a brief, standardised method by which to grade cognitive mental status. It assesses orientation, attention, immediate and short-term recall, language, and the ability to follow simple verbal and written commands. Scoring allows the individual to be rated as to cognitive function, and the results of successive tests to be compared over time.

The abbreviated mental test score (AMT) is a quick way to evaluate cognitive function in general practice to screen for dementia or monitor its progression.[5] The AMT consists of a set of 10 questions for the patient and takes about 10 minutes to administer and complete (*see* Box 7.2). A cognitively intact person should answer the 10 questions correctly, whereas a score below 6 indicates likely cognitive impairment.

Box 7.2:   The abbreviated mental test score[5]

Each correct answer scores one point

 1   Age
 2   Time to nearest hour
 3   An address to be repeated by the patient at the end of the test
 4   Year
 5   Name of hospital or residence etc where patient is situated
 6   Recognition of two persons e.g. doctor, home help, etc
 7   Date of birth
 8   Year that the First World War started
 9   Name of present monarch
10   Count backwards from 20 to 1

The 6CIT consists of six questions that are simple and non-cultural and do not require any complex interpretation (*see* Box 7.3). GPs have found that the 6CIT is more appropriate for those with mild dementia than the MMSE.[6] The 6CIT can be loaded on the practice computer as a Windows-based program.[11]

Box 7.3:   The 6CIT test

Try to perform the test in a quiet place with no obvious clock or calendar visible to the patient. Score the test as in the list below.

- Ask question 1 and then question 2 (*see* below).
- Tell the patient you are going to tell them a fictional address which you would like them to try to memorise and then repeat back to you afterwards. Say the address. Make sure the patient is able to repeat the address correctly before moving on and warn them to try to memorise it as you are going to ask them to repeat it again in a few minutes. No score is made at this stage.
- Ask the patient the time, if they get within 60 minutes of the correct time then they score 0, if not then score 3.
- Ask the patient to count backwards from 20 to 1. If they do this correctly score 0. If they make one error score 2; two or more errors score 4.
- Ask the patient to say the months of the year backwards starting with December. Give them plenty of time for this and it doesn't matter if they keep saying the months forward in order to get the answer.
- Finally ask them to repeat the address back to you. The address is broken into five fragments and is scored for each error (*see* list below).

1   What year is it?   Correct 0; incorrect 4
2   What month is it?   Correct 0; incorrect 3
3   Remember the following address: John Brown, 42 West Street, Bedford

4	What time is it?	Correct 0; incorrect 3
5	Count backwards from 20 to 1	Correct 0; one error 2; more than one error 4
6	Say the months of the year backwards	Correct 0; one error 2; more than one error 4
7	Repeat memory phrase	Correct 0; one error 2; two errors 4; three errors 6; four errors 8; all incorrect 10

Interpreting the score

0–7: normal

8–9: mild cognitive impairment – refer to memory clinic

10–28: significant cognitive impairment

The Clifton Assessment Procedures for the Elderly (CAPE) are useful to give a profile for a patient but do not provide a score.[2,12] It is quick and easy to fill in together with observations from carers (*see* Box 7.4). It can be used to estimate the likelihood of strain on the carer.

Box 7.4: The Clifton Assessment Procedures for the Elderly (CAPE)[2,12]

Information/orientation

- Can you give me your name?
- Can you tell the name of where you are now?
- Who is the prime minister now?
- What day is it?
- Can you give me your address?
- Can you tell the address of where you are now?
- Who is the president of the United States?
- What month is it?
- Can you tell me your date of birth?
- Can you tell the name of the town/city where you are now?
- What colour is the flag?
- What year is it?

Physical disability

- When bathing or dressing, he/she requires:
  - no help
  - some help
  - maximum help
- With regard to walking, he/she:
  - shows no signs of weakness
  - walks slowly without aid, or uses a stick

- is unable to walk (or if able to walk needs a frame, crutches or someone by their side)
- He/she is incontinent of urine and/or faeces (day or night):
  - never
  - sometimes (once or twice a week)
  - frequently (three times a week or more)
- He/she is in bed during the day (bed does not include couch, settee etc):
  - never
  - sometimes
  - almost always
- He/she is confused (unable to find way around, loses possessions etc):
  - almost never
  - sometimes
  - almost always
- Left to his/her own devices, his/her appearance (clothes and/or hair) is:
  - almost never disorderly
  - sometimes disorderly
  - almost always disorderly

Some areas have memory clinics – of which some see only patients at an early stage of dementia, and others perform multidisciplinary assessments at any stage of dementia. You should know if there is a clinic near you and what are the criteria for referral.[2]

The importance of early diagnosis[13]

Early diagnosis allows the patient and family to plan for the future and identify outside sources of assistance. As potentially useful and proven treatments become available, early diagnosis of dementia will become increasingly important. Although screening all elderly patients for dementia is not warranted, being alert for cognitive and functional decline is a prudent way of recognising dementia in its early stage. Knowing the diagnosis provides carers with an explanation for their relative's behaviour and stops them from blaming themselves or the relative.

In addition, early detection may lead to the detection and treatment of co-existing medical conditions that can be mistaken for dementia or that may be contributing to its severity.

The primary care team has a central role in the diagnosis and ongoing care of dementia. Its roles in diagnosis and management include:

- identifying people who have suspected dementia
- excluding treatable causes

- referring to specialist psychiatric services when the diagnosis is uncertain
- providing information about the diagnosis and prognosis of dementia
- assessing the informal carer's ability to cope
- providing information about available services and benefits
- helping with access to, and co-ordination of, a range of support services
- providing emotional support to informal carers
- treating co-existing conditions as they occur
- monitoring and co-ordinating care of the individual with dementia
- prescribing new drugs for dementia in association with the physician initiating treatment.

Classification of dementia[14]

Dementia is classified as minimal, mild, moderate or severe dementia. Each stage merges into the next one. Dementia may be temporarily worse with intercurrent illness.

Minimal dementia

A person with 'minimal' dementia has some difficulty in recalling recent events and may be prone to mislaying or losing things. A person with minimal dementia is usually still independent and care is probably not needed.

Mild dementia

A person with 'mild' dementia has most or all of the following signs and symptoms:

- difficulty in recalling recent information
- limited or patchy disorientation in time and place
- impaired problem solving, reasoning and the ability to manage everyday activities.

In the later stages of mild dementia, some degree of care will usually be required.

Moderate dementia

A person with 'moderate' dementia has most of the following signs and symptoms:

- severely impaired reasoning, problem solving and recall of recent events
- disorientated in time and place

- speech slightly unclear, but not to a marked degree
- not able to manage housework, shopping and finances independently
- needs help with dressing and other self-care
- may be occasionally incontinent.

Daily care is usually required for those with moderate dementia.

Severe dementia

A person with 'severe' dementia:

- is totally disorientated
- is incapable of recall, reasoning and self-care
- is unable to communicate in normal speech
- may fail to recognise close relatives
- is almost invariably incontinent, apathetic and inert.

The person with severe dementia may become immobile, and will be totally incapable of being independent. Continual care and supervision are usually required.

The need for care depends on how long an individual can remain living alone or being independent. The needs of an individual tend to vary from time to time, as there may be episodes of severely disturbed behaviour. Health and social care services need to be flexible.

Case study 7.1 continued

Mrs Grey telephones you to say that Mr Grey has agreed to attend for a 'well-man' check with the practice nurse. You brief the practice nurse who has been trained in administering the 6CIT loaded on the computer. You arrange for Mr Grey to have some screening blood and urine tests and to see you for the results following his 'well-man' check. The results suggest that he has mild dementia, with some awareness of his decline in ability, and is depressed. Mr Grey agrees to be referred to the memory clinic, as there might be a possibility of receiving treatment initiated by the specialist. In the meantime, he agrees to try an antidepressant and to see you again about this in a couple of weeks. You suggest Mrs Grey contacts Age Concern[15] or the Alzheimer's Society[2] so that she can start making some longer-term plans.

Treatment of dementia

The North of England evidence-based guidelines development project and SIGN give similar recommendations for pharmacological treatments.[16,17] Neuroleptic drugs are the mainstay of pharmacological treatment for Alzheimer's disease but they do have side-effects such as parkinsonism, drowsiness, tardive dyskinesia, falls accelerating cognitive decline, and severe neuroleptic sensitivity reactions. Patients with dementia from Lewy bodies are more sensitive to the side-effects of neuroleptic medication and should not be prescribed these medications, so an accurate diagnosis is imperative.[16]

NICE recommendations about donepezil, rivastigmine and galantamine in the treatment of Alzheimer's disease are shown in Box 7.5.[18]

Box 7.5: NICE recommendations for treatment with donepezil, rivastigmine and galantamine in Alzheimer's disease[18]

1 Diagnosis that the form of dementia is AD must be made in a specialist clinic according to standard diagnostic criteria.

2 Assessment in a specialist clinic, including tests of cognitive, global and behavioural functioning and of activities of daily living, should be made before the drug is prescribed.

3 Clinicians should exercise judgement about the likelihood of compliance; in general, a carer or care-worker who is in sufficient contact with the patient to ensure compliance should be a minimum requirement.

4 Only specialists (including old age psychiatrists, neurologists, and care of the elderly physicians) should initiate treatment.

5 Carers' views of the patient's condition at baseline and follow-up should be sought. If GPs are to take over prescribing, it is recommended that they should do so under an agreed shared-care protocol with clear treatment endpoints.

6 A further assessment should be made, usually two to four months after reaching a maintenance dose of the drug. Following this assessment the drug should be continued only where there has been an improvement or no deterioration in MMSE score, together with evidence of global improvement on the basis of behavioural and/or functional assessment.

7 Patients who continue on the drug should be reviewed by MMSE score and global, functional and behavioural assessment every six months. The drug should normally only be continued while their MMSE score remains above 12 points, and their global, functional and behavioural condition remains at a level where the drug is considered to be having a worthwhile effect. When the MMSE score falls below 12 points, patients should not normally be prescribed any of these drugs. Any review involving MMSE assessment should be undertaken by an appropriate specialist team, unless there are locally agreed protocols for shared care.

Treatment with olanzapine, risperidone or carbamazepine has been tried if agitation, delusions or hallucinations are present.[3] The adverse effects of atypical antipsychotic drugs, particularly in increasing the tendency to fall and the incidence of diabetes, means that non-pharmaceutical measures should be tried first. Moreover, recent evidence about the increased risk of mortality and stroke in people treated with olanzapine has prompted a change in recommendations. Olanzapine is now not approved for the treatment of dementia-related psychosis.[19]

Low-dose aspirin (75–150 mg daily) may be indicated in MID.

Mr and Mrs Grey will want to discuss what they can do themselves while awaiting the decision at the memory clinic. Clinical evidence evaluates the following treatments as beneficial.[3]

* An extract of ginkgo biloba, taken as a 40 mg tablet three times daily before food, seems to be effective for people with dementia and is well tolerated. The 'number needed to treat' (NNT) calculation predicts that about seven patients with dementia have to be treated with 120 mg of ginkgo extract daily for one year for one of them to have an improvement which they would not have had with placebo treatment. That level of improvement is equivalent to a six-month delay in the progression of the dementia.[20]
* There seems to be an association between high levels of serum homocysteine and low levels of serum folate and dementia. The conclusion of one review was that taking a daily multivitamin is likely to prevent cardiovascular disease, cancer and possibly dementia.[21]
* Reality orientation presents the patient with orientation information through techniques such as the use of calendars, cueing, and reinforcement by repetition of information, and is thought to provide the patient with a greater understanding of his or her environment (*see* Box 7.6).

Box 7.6:   Reality orientation

* Surround people with Alzheimer's disease with familiar objects that can be used to stimulate their memory. Other materials, such as a family scrapbook, flash cards, Scrabble games, a globe, large-piece jigsaw puzzles, and illustrated, large-print dictionaries, also help.
* Another tool, the reality-orientation board, is any board with a surface on which information can be changed easily, such as a blackboard, a pegboard, or an erasable memo board. Both the caregiver and the person with Alzheimer's disease fill in information such as current day of the week, date, and year, and the weather.
* For persons who are severely confused, the focus is on less complicated information, such as their own name and address, the name of their caregiver, colours, and identification of everyday objects.

- Reality orientation is around-the-clock therapy; the caregiver and anyone should be encouraged to apply the techniques. General guidelines include the following:
    - treat people with memory impairment with respect. Do not talk down to them or treat them like children
    - every conversation you have with the person should include mention of the time, day of the week, and names of familiar people and objects.

People with Alzheimer's should be encouraged to perform activities of daily living, that is, getting dressed, eating and taking care of personal hygiene, and should be complimented on all such attempts.

Other forms of therapy have unknown effectiveness and are still under review. Reminiscence work and music therapy are unlikely to harm and may make Mrs Grey and her family feel that they are contributing to Mr Grey's care in a positive way. The Alzheimer's Association will be able to keep Mrs Grey up to date on the latest information.[2]

Collecting data to demonstrate your learning, competence, performance and standards of service delivery

Example cycle of evidence 7.1

- Focus: relationships with patients
- Other relevant foci: maintaining good medical practice; working with colleagues; probity

Stages of the evidence cycle

Stage 1
Select targets

Stage 2
Set standards

Stage 5
Document it all

Stage 3A/B
Identify needs

Stage 4
Learning/action plan

Case study 7.2

Mrs French requests a visit for her husband. Your partner, who usually sees Mr French, is away on a course. The receptionist tells you that usually Mr French, who has Alzheimer's disease, rings demanding a visit for various ailments that he has forgotten are all being treated. He is on medication for prostate problems and osteoarthritis. Usually when the surgery rings back, Mrs French says wearily that he has no new problems and not to bother. Mrs French does much valuable work with the local branch of the Alzheimer's Association and has mobilised all possible assistance for her husband. This time when you ring, she explains that her brother-in-law is visiting from France and is insisting on a visit, as he believes she and your GP partner have been ignoring his requests for help.

When you attend, the brother-in-law and Mr French are quite intimidating. The brother-in-law tells you that he was not aware of his brother's deteriorating function and tells you that you must immediately prescribe for him. He has written down a list of drugs that are, as he puts it, 'essential'. The list includes galantamine, ginkgo biloba, folic acid and trazodone. You try to explain that Mr French had been on donepezil, but had shown no improvement, so it had been stopped. The brother-in-law brushes aside your explanations as 'money-saving'. You find yourself uncomfortably agreeing to ask the specialist to review him, although you know that the waiting list is long and he will not have any priority as he has already been assessed. You can see Mrs French behind the two of them, shaking her head at you.

This is just an example. Keep your task simple. You could choose three or four cycles of evidence to demonstrate your competence each year.

Stage 1: Select your aspirations for good practice

The excellent GP:

- seeks consent before sharing information
- provides or arranges investigations or treatment when necessary
- refers to another practitioner when indicated
- keeps open lines of communication with colleagues
- works with colleagues to monitor and maintain the quality of care provided
- makes sure that others understand his professional status and speciality, what roles and responsibilities he has and who is responsible for each aspect of the patient's care.

Stage 2: Set the standards for your outcomes

Outcomes might include:

- the way learning is applied
- a learnt skill
- a protocol
- a strategy that is implemented
- meeting recommended standards.

- Demonstrate consistent best practice in the management of patients with dementia.
- Document best practice in managing the concerns of relatives and seeking consent for the sharing of information.

Stage 3A: Identify your learning needs

- Self-assess your knowledge about the NICE guidelines for treatment with galantamine.[18]
- Keep a reflective diary about how you handled your irritation over the relative's assumption that you, your partner and Mrs French were providing inadequate care.
- Think how best to obtain consent to disclosure of medical information when a patient is accompanied by a relative and has cognitive deficiencies.

Stage 3B: Identify your service needs

> Any of the needs assessment exercises in 3A may also reveal service needs.

- Look at the practice guidelines for review of patients with dementia.
- Review the practice policy for managing requests for referral to a specialist when the health professional is not the usual one who is caring for the patient.

Stage 4: Make and carry out a learning and action plan

- Read up on the current NICE guidelines[18] and the evidence in *Clinical Evidence Concise*.[3]
- Discuss the practice guidelines for review of patients with dementia at a practice meeting.
- Attend workshops on best practice on consent to disclosure of medical information and managing the concerns of relatives.
- Discuss with colleagues how to manage requests for referral from relatives, and requests to health professionals not usually responsible for the care of that patient.

Stage 5: Document your learning, competence, performance and standards of service delivery

- Keep a copy of the practice guidelines for review of patients with dementia.

- Include feedback from other health professionals about how they manage requests for referral from relatives, and to health professionals not usually responsible for the care of that patient.
- Keep your notes from the workshops on best practice on consent to disclosure of medical information and managing the concerns of relatives.

Case study 7.2 continued

You ask one of the receptionists, who lives near Mrs French, to drop round a copy of the patient information from the NICE recommendations,[18] together with a printout of the latest information from *Clinical Evidence Concise*[3] for her brother-in-law to read that evening. The following day, you discuss Mr French's management with your partner, who points out that Mr French had had an extended appointment to review all his ailments in the surgery only two months previously. Your partner thinks that a family conference with the sons and daughter who live nearer and visit more often may be required to prevent interference from a relative who has not seen his brother for several years. He will discuss this with Mrs French.

The procedure for review of patients with dementia by the practice team is found to be working well and does not require any change.

Following the workshops on managing the concerns of relatives and obtaining consent from patients with cognitive impairment, you feel more confident that you will manage this type of consultation better in future.

Example cycle of evidence 7.2

- Focus: clinical care
- Other relevant foci: working with colleagues; relationships with patients; management

Stages of the evidence cycle
Stage 1
Select targets
Stage 2
Set standards
Stage 5
Document it all
Stage 3A/B
Identify needs
Stage 4
Learning/action plan

Case study 7.3

Dr Script is the prescribing lead for a large group practice. She returns from a meeting to find an email on the internal system from the practice manager, informing her that there has been a safety warning about olanzapine in the mail the previous day. She sifts through the pile of unread mail in her in-tray. The notification recommends that elderly patients being treated for dementia-related psychosis and/or behavioural disturbances should have their treatment reviewed and discussed with them and/or their carers.[19] She will have to take some action.

This is just an example. Keep your task simple. You could choose three or four cycles of evidence to demonstrate your competence each year.

Stage 1: Select your aspirations for good practice

The excellent GP:

- has a structured approach for managing long-term health problems and preventive care
- responds rapidly to new information
- reviews medication in the light of new research.

Stage 2: Set the standards for your outcomes

> Outcomes might include:
>
> - the way learning is applied
> - a learnt skill
> - a protocol
> - a strategy that is implemented
> - meeting recommended standards.

- Patients with a confirmed diagnosis of dementia have a Read code entry to that effect.
- The prescribing information for atypical antipsychotics is modified on the system.
- All of the practice team are aware of the change.

Stage 3A: Identify your learning needs

- Self-assess your knowledge of the indications and contraindications for treatment with olanzapine and other atypical antipsychotics.
- Review the evidence for the effects and harms of treatments for the behavioural and psychological symptoms of dementia, with the attached community psychiatric nurse.

Stage 3B: Identify your service needs

> Any of the needs assessment exercises in 3A may also reveal service needs.

- Establish how other practice team members are recording the diagnosis of dementia.

- Arrange for a computer search and printout of practice patients for the combination of prescriptions of atypical antipsychotics and the diagnosis of dementia.

Stage 4: Make and carry out a learning and action plan

- Arrange to give a presentation on dementia treatments, together with the attached community psychiatric nurse at a practice meeting. You give the information about indications and contraindications for treatment with olanzapine and other atypical antipsychotics, and the evidence for the effects and harms of treatments for the behavioural and psychological symptoms of dementia.
- Discuss at the practice meeting the support that team members, patients and carers might need in altering established treatments.
- Arrange who will contact the patients/carers of each patient on the list of patients with dementia who are receiving atypical antipsychotic medication.
- Discuss with the practice team whether to be more cautious in the use of atypical antipsychotic medication in elderly patients.

Stage 5: Document your learning, competence, performance and standards of service delivery

- Print out the search of practice patients for the combination of prescriptions of atypical antipsychotic medication and the diagnosis of dementia again in three months time, to ensure that the proposed action has taken place.
- Record the steps taken to provide support for team members, patients and carers affected by the change.
- Record the changes to the drug information for atypical antipsychotic medication provided on the computer.
- Record the way in which an automatic email will alert the attached community psychiatric nurse so that she obtains early warning of possible problems with the use of atypical antipsychotic medication in the elderly and can inform the practice team.

Case study 7.3 continued

Fortunately, only a few patients with dementia were taking olanzapine. Some of these had to be referred back to the psychogeriatrician for further advice on their management. Dr Script set up a similar search for other atypical antipsychotics in patients over the age of 65 years. She arranged for the records to be flagged for their medication to be reviewed in view of the concerns of an increased risk of stroke or mortality in patients with other risk factors such as dysphagia, sedation or concomitant use of benzodiazepines, or pulmonary conditions.

Example cycle of evidence 7.3

- Focus: teaching and training
- Other relevant foci: relationships with patients and carers; maintaining good medical practice

---

Case study 7.4

A medical student is sitting in your surgery when Miss Wisp arrives with her neighbour Mrs Worthy. Miss Wisp says that she just gets anxious, and is just a bit forgetful nowadays. Mrs Worthy takes over and explains that she pops in to keep an eye on her 68-year-old neighbour. Miss Wisp seems fine one day but 'totally with the fairies' on another day. She reminds Miss Wisp of various episodes recently – putting on her clothes over her nightie, burning out a saucepan that she put empty onto the cooking ring, spending hours looking for her keys or her glasses that she thinks have been hidden by someone who has come into the house, forgetting to pay bills and not eating properly. Miss Wisp breaks down in tears and says she doesn't understand why she cannot cope some days. Her niece has stopped coming to see her after she accused Miss Wisp of playing at being helpless to get attention. You ask if the medical student can do a memory test and Miss Wisp manages the abbreviated mental test score with only one error. The student says 'I don't think there's much wrong with your memory' and Miss Wisp looks as if she will burst into tears again. You intervene to arrange some investigations and ask to see her again – you suggest she attends on a 'not-good' day to assess her again and Mrs Worthy agrees to bring her again.

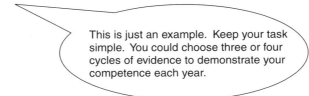

This is just an example. Keep your task simple. You could choose three or four cycles of evidence to demonstrate your competence each year.

Stage 1: Select your aspirations for good practice

The excellent GP:

- helps to educate other colleagues at all levels
- does not undermine the confidence of juniors or students
- treats patients with courtesy and consideration
- keeps his/her knowledge up to date.

Stage 2: Set the standards for your outcomes

Outcomes might include:

- the way learning is applied
- a learnt skill
- a protocol
- a strategy that is implemented
- meeting recommended standards.

- Demonstrate an active involvement in the training of another.
- Behave in a courteous way to patients and students.
- Be up to date with knowledge about dementia.

Stage 3A: Identify your learning needs

- Review your teaching skills by obtaining consent to videotape a tutorial with the medical student and exchanging videos with another trainer for mutual peer review.
- Check that your knowledge about dementia is correct and up to date by checking against best practice.
- Obtain feedback from the students, anonymised via the medical school.
- Check whether you have the skills to guide the student to manage this type of problem.

Stage 3B: Identify your service needs

> Any of the needs assessment exercises in 3A may also reveal service needs.

- Find out what help the health visitor and district nurse can give the medical student to learn about how patients with dementia can be helped to manage at home, and what options are available if they cannot manage at home.
- Ask the practice nurse who supervises the provision of patient literature to review with the medical student the usefulness of the literature on dementia available in the practice to patients and carers.

Stage 4: Make and carry out a learning and action plan

- Read about dementia, and particularly about the diagnosis of Lewy Body dementia (LBD).
- Prepare and give a tutorial for the medical student on the diagnosis and management of dementia.
- Attend a refresher course for teachers and trainers.
- Read the literature on dementia, selected as most useful by the medical student and practice nurse, so that you can recommend it appropriately to patients and carers.

Stage 5: Document your learning, competence, performance and standards of service delivery

- Keep a record of the results of the peer review of your tutorial and feedback from students.
- Record your new knowledge about dementia.
- Keep a list of the available selected patient information literature on dementia.
- Keep your notes of the teachers' and trainers' course.

Case study 7.4 continued

You give a tutorial to the medical student with your new knowledge. You learn some more from the work the medical student has done to find out the literature available to patients with dementia and their carers. The medical student is amazed at the complexity of the job the GP is expected to do, and acknowledges that she was less than tactful telling Miss Wisp that there was nothing wrong with her memory when she hears about the variable nature of the cognitive changes in Lewy Body dementia.

> You have a more appropriate supply of literature for patients with dementia and their carers. You feel that your teaching skills have been improved by the attendance at the course and the reviews and reflections about the task.

References

1 Erikinjuntti T, Østbye T, Steenhuis R *et al.* (1997) The effect of different diagnostic criteria on the prevalence of dementia. *New England Journal of Medicine.* **337:** 1667–74.

2 Alzheimer's Disease Association: www.alzheimers.org.uk

3 Godlee F (ed.) (2004) *Clinical Evidence Concise.* Issue 11. BMJ Publishing Group, London. www.clinicalevidence.com

4 Thistlethwaite J (2000) Dementia: the role of the primary care team. *Update.* **17 August:** 150–4.

5 Folstein MF, Folstein SE and McHugh PR (1975) Mini-mental state: a practical method for grading the cognitive state of patients for the clinician. *Journal of Psychiatric Research.* **12:** 189–98.

6 Foord-Kelcey G (ed.) (2004) Diagnosis and management of dementia in primary care. *Guidelines.* **22:** 143–4. www.eguidelines.co.uk

7 Research Unit of the Royal College of Physicians and the British Geriatrics Society (1992) *Standardised Assessment Scales for Elderly People.* The Royal College of Physicians of London and the British Geriatrics Society, London.

8 Brooke P and Bullock R (1999) Validation of the 6 item cognitive impairment test. *International Journal of Geriatric Psychiatry.* **14:** 936–40.

9 Brooke P (2000) A better test for cognitive loss. *The Practitioner.* **244:** 389 and 463.

10 Sunderland T, Hill JL, Mellow AM *et al.* (1989) Clock drawing in Alzheimer's disease. A novel measure of dementia severity. *Journal of the American Geriatric Society.* **37:** 725–9.

11 www.kingshill-research.org/kresearch/6cit.asp

12 www.ehr.chime.ucl.ac.uk/demcare/cape.html

13 Iliffe S, Manthorpe J and Eden A (2003) Sooner or later? Issues in the early diagnosis of dementia in general practice: a qualitative study. *Family Practice.* **20(4):** 376–81.

14 Audit Commission (2000) *Forget Me Not – mental health services for older people.* Audit Commission, London.

15 www.ageconcern.org.uk

16   Eccles M, Clarke J and Livingston M (1998) North of England evidence-based guidelines development project: guideline for the primary care management of dementia. *British Medical Journal.* **317:** 802–8.

17   Scottish Intercollegiate Guidelines Network (1998) *Interventions in the Management of Behavioural and Psychological Aspects of Dementia.* Scottish Intercollegiate Guidelines Network, Edinburgh. www.sign.ac.uk

18   Technology Appraisal Guidance (2003) *Guidance on the Use of Donepezil, Rivastigmine and Galantamine for the Treatment of Alzheimer's Disease.* National Institute for Clinical Evidence, London. www.nice.org.uk

19   www.emea.eu.int/htms/human/drugalert/drugalert.htm

20   Moore A, McQuay H and Muir Gray JA (1998) Dementia diagnosis and treatment. *Bandolier.* **5(2):** 2–3.

21   Moore A, McQuay H and Muir Gray JA (1999) Folate, homocysteine and dementia. *Bandolier.* **6(9):** 1–2.

8

Diabetes

There are four subcategories of diabetes:

* type 1
* type 2
* gestational
* other specific types e.g. drug-induced.

In people with type 1 diabetes, the pancreas is no longer able to produce insulin because the insulin-producing cells (the beta-cells) have been destroyed by the body's immune system.

In type 2 diabetes, the beta-cells are not able to produce enough insulin for the body's needs – and in addition, the majority of people with type 2 diabetes have some degree of resistance to insulin.[1,2]

Gestational diabetes describes the 'carbohydrate intolerance of variable severity with onset or first recognition in pregnancy' that occurs in 2–4% of pregnancies in the UK.[3]

Other specific types include:

* genetic defects of beta-cell function
* genetic defects in insulin action
* diseases of the pancreas (e.g. pancreatitis)
* endocrinopathies (e.g. acromegaly)
* drug- or chemical-induced diabetes (e.g. caused by thiazides, steroids)
* infections (e.g. congenital rubella)
* uncommon forms of immune-mediated diabetes (e.g. due to anti-insulin antibodies)
* other genetic syndromes sometimes associated with diabetes (e.g. Down's syndrome).

Type 2 diabetes mellitus

Case study 8.1

Mrs Waite is a 56 year old who came to see you two weeks ago complaining of being 'tired all the time'. She had no other symptoms, and you advised her about tackling her obesity and smoking habit. You organised blood tests for a full blood count, thyroid function and plasma glucose. When the glucose concentration came back at 12.3 mmol/l, you arranged for her to have a fasting blood glucose test. This was 8.4 mmol/l. She is not surprised by your diagnosis of diabetes, as her mother took tablets for diabetes, which she developed in her 50s too. Her mother died of a stroke aged 70 years.

What issues you should cover

You should tell Mrs Waite about diabetes, so that she knows to take her condition seriously. Tell her that diabetes mellitus is caused by a raised blood glucose concentration (hyperglycaemia) due to insufficient insulin, or the presence of factors opposing its action. It is a chronic, progressive disease which can result in premature death, ill-health and disability. Emphasise to Mrs Waite that the consequences of diabetes can be prevented or delayed by high quality care and her taking control and managing her condition in line with the best advice and treatment.

Definition

Definitions vary. The World Health Organization's (WHO's) definition of diabetes is: 'diabetes mellitus describes a metabolic disorder of multiple aetiology characterised by chronic hyperglycaemia with disturbances of carbohydrate, fat and protein metabolism resulting from defects in insulin secretion, insulin action or both.'[4] A current definition is fasting plasma glucose ≥ 7.0 mmol/l, or ≥ 11.1 mmol/l two hours after 75 g oral glucose load, on two or more occasions.[5,6]

Insulin resistance distinguishes type 2 from type 1 diabetes. Insulin resistance occurs when the body fails to respond to its own normally circulating insulin so that there is less of a blood glucose-lowering effect. At first the body compensates by producing more insulin from the pancreas. But less insulin is eventually produced as the beta-cells of the pancreas become exhausted. A person with type 2 diabetes typically has reduced insulin secretion coupled with insulin resistance in the liver, adipose tissue and skeletal muscle, leading to a loss of control of blood glucose.

One cause of insulin resistance is thought to be the dumping of surplus fat around the abdomen in preference to other parts of the body. The genetic make-up of people prone to insulin resistance encourages them to store surplus energy as abdominal fat rather than glycogen in skeletal muscle. This 'apple' shaped human form is more likely to convey a risk of early death from heart disease as opposed to a 'pear' shaped form. Avoiding obesity and being physically active reduces the risks and effects of insulin resistance.

Prevalence

Between 2% and 3% of people of all ages in the UK have type 1 or type 2 diabetes.[7] About 200 000 people are thought to have type 1 and more than a million have type 2 diabetes.[8] More than 95 000 new cases of type 2 diabetes are diagnosed each year in the UK. There are another million adults in the UK who are thought to have type 2 diabetes which is not, as yet, diagnosed. In a population of 100 000 people, between 2000 and 3000 would be known to have diabetes, of whom approximately 25–30 will be children.[1] The lifetime risk for a person living in the UK developing type 2 diabetes is probably greater than 10%.[8]

In the UK, type 2 diabetes is up to six times more common in adults of South Asian descent and up to three times more common in people of African and African–Caribbean origins, compared with the white population. Diabetes is also more common in people of Chinese descent and other non-white groups. But there is little difference in prevalence between children from various ethnic groups. Up to one-fifth of over-25-year-old Asians and African–Caribbean people living in the UK may have type 2 diabetes.[1,8]

The prevalence of diabetes mellitus increases with age. As many as one in 20 people over the age of 65 years and one in five over the age of 85 years in the UK has type 2 diabetes.[1,8] Diabetes is more common in people from the most deprived section of the population in the UK, and diabetes complications are several times more likely in people with diabetes from social class V compared with those from social class I.[1]

Diagnosis

Mrs Waite has type 2 diabetes. When you question her, she has the early symptoms of type 2 diabetes: tiredness, blurred vision, increasing thirst, weight loss and passing urine more often. Like Mrs Waite, many people with non-diagnosed diabetes may put down the symptoms at first to be due to increasing age. Because of this delay in presenting, half of those that are newly diagnosed with diabetes may already have early signs of complications.

Case study 8.1 continued

You explain to Mrs Waite that the raised fasting blood glucose level confirms that she has diabetes. You check that she has not been taking any other drugs that might have precipitated diabetes (*see* page 159). You assess Mrs Waite's cardiovascular risks. You already know that she is a smoker and you examine her physically, assessing her cardiovascular system and looking for complications of diabetes. You arrange for her to have a prolonged consultation with the nurse practitioner who is the lead for diabetes in the practice. She does a thorough baseline assessment of Mrs Waite's lifestyle, taking time to explain the nature of diabetes and the aims of treatment. She undertakes further blood tests according to your practice protocol for patients with newly diagnosed diabetes.

Initial management of people with newly diagnosed type 2 diabetes[1,6,9]

Initial discussion should include:

- the history of illness, looking for underlying causes or complications of diabetes
- a simple explanation of diabetes, responding to questions and anxieties
- a discussion of lifestyle: smoking, diet, exercise, alcohol intake
- an explanation of the practice organisation and different roles of the primary healthcare team and how to obtain advice as needed
- information about Diabetes UK, how to access it and how it will help.

Examination should include:

- calculation of body mass index (BMI) from weight and height measurement
- blood pressure
- full clinical examination to exclude underlying causes of diabetes such as pancreatic disease, and make an assessment of any existing complications of diabetes.

Investigations may include (this list will vary according to local guidance):

- urinanalysis for glucose, ketones and protein (subsequent midstream urinanalysis if microalbuminuria is detected)
- fasting plasma glucose (as already described above)
- full blood count
- haemoglobin A_{1c} (HbA_{1c})
- renal profile
- liver function tests
- fasting lipid profile
- thyroid function tests.

Initial management should include:

- referral to a diabetes specialist if the patient is unwell (e.g. has marked recent weight loss), if there is ketonuria, or if the blood glucose concentration is >20 mmol/l. If patients are reasonably well, like Mrs Waite, they can have a trial of controlling the diabetes with dietary measures for three months
- initial dietary assessment and advice
- referral to a dietitian or member of a specialist diabetes team such as a community diabetes educator if indicated and if available
- referral to a podiatrist or chiropodist, and optometrist if necessary
- discussion and agreement of an individualised management plan with targets as appropriate: including change to a healthy balanced diet, restriction of refined sugars and alcohol, increasing exercise, stopping smoking – as appropriate
- making a follow-up appointment
- entering the patient on the practice diabetes register and recall system; recording the patient on the district diabetes register if one exists.

Management of patients with type 2 diabetes

There are two main aims of treatment for diabetes:

1. to allow as normal a daily life as possible without symptoms, while at the same time avoiding acute complications such as ketoacidosis, hypoglycaemia and infection
2. to prevent or delay the long-term specific complications of diabetes including microangiopathy (retinopathy, nephropathy), cataract and neuropathy, and to decrease the excess morbidity and mortality from macrovascular disease.[10]

A key outcome measure of good diabetes management is blood glucose control, as measured by how low the levels are of glycated haemoglobin (HbA$_{1c}$). This indicates the quality of blood glucose control over the preceding two to three months. The target should reflect individual circumstances, aiming between 6.5% and 7.5%.[11]

Other helpful outcome measures include: pre-and post-meal blood glucose levels, the extent to which acute episodes of hypoglycaemia and hyperglycaemia are prevented, and reduction in macrovascular risk factors such as raised blood pressure, smoking, obesity and dyslipidaemia.[11]

The review of patients with type 2 diabetes includes the indicators covered by the quality and outcomes indicators of the GMS contract. In brief, reviews should be at least annual and include:

- information about blood glucose levels contributed by self-monitoring by the patient (the frequency should depend on how good average control is)
- a chat to the patient about their wellbeing, e.g. eliciting sensitive problems such as impotence
- calculation of BMI and noting whether it is rising or reducing
- recording lifestyle habits: smoking status, whether ceased smoking or advised to quit
- recording blood pressure at least annually: aiming for a blood pressure of less than 140/80 mmHg. Initiate antihypertensive treatment if systolic blood pressure is sustained at or over 140 mmHg or diastolic blood pressure is sustained at or over 90 mmHg. Aim for an optimal blood pressure goal of 130/80 mmHg or less for patients with diabetes on antihypertensive treatment.[12] In those with microalbuminuria or proteinuria, aim to achieve a target blood pressure of 135/75 mmHg or less
- checking a midstream urine sample for proteinuria. If it is positive, send off a midstream urine for analysis to detect infection. Treat if appropriate, and repeat the check for proteinuria. Arrange a 24-hour collection of urine for protein and creatinine clearance. If protein levels in the urine are more than 0.3 g per 24 h refer to a diabetic nephrologist
- checking for microalbuminuria with a dip stick or sending early morning urine to the lab to test for albumin or an albumin/creatinine ratio. Repeat positive tests on at least two more occasions over the next six months and repeat a negative test annually. If positive, the patient should be started on an angiotensin converting enzyme (ACE) inhibitor or angiotensin-2 (A2) antagonist to prevent progression of diabetic nephropathy. Patients' records of their annual test for microalbuminuria should be coded separately if the patient has existing proteinuria, when claiming quality points for the quality outcomes framework
- recording any retinopathy, noting if retinal photography has been undertaken: ophthalmoscopy should be performed by an appropriately trained GP, specialist or local optometrist
- foot examination by appropriately trained professional (podiatrist): test foot sensation using a 10 g monofilament or vibration, palpate foot pulses, inspect any foot deformity and footwear. Patients should be classified as low current risk, at increased risk, at high risk or having an ulcerated foot. Those at increased risk with a neuropathy or absent pulses should be reviewed at 3–6-monthly intervals. Those at high risk with a neuropathy and absent pulses together with deformity or skin changes or previous ulcer should be seen 1–3 monthly by the foot protection team. In any foot care

emergency such as new ulceration, swelling or discoloration, the patient should be referred to the multidisciplinary foot care team within 24 h[13]
- blood tests: HbA_{1c} (aim for less than 7.5%); fasting serum cholesterol (aim for 5.0 mmol/l or below) plus low-density (LDL) and high-density lipoproteins (HDL) and triglycerides; serum creatinine (if raised refer to nephrologists – the rate of rise triggering referral will depend on local protocol)
- reinforcing patient education.

See *Diabetes Matters in Primary Care*[2] for more detailed information.

Overview of medication for patients with type 2 diabetes

BIGUANIDES (E.G. METFORMIN)

Metformin is the drug of first choice in overweight patients in whom strict dieting has failed to control their blood glucose levels. It is also used in patients who are not overweight or are inadequately controlled with a sulphonylurea drug.[14] Biguanides lower blood glucose by inhibiting hepatic glucose production. Start with a low dose (e.g. 500 mg per day for at least a week) before increasing the dose gradually in order to help combat gastrointestinal intolerance. Adverse effects are common and include gastrointestinal symptoms, and, rarely, lactic acidosis. Avoid using metformin in people with heart failure, or in kidney or liver failure and alcoholism.

SULPHONYLUREAS (E.G. GLIBENCLAMIDE, GLICLAZIDE, GLIMEPIRIDE, GLIPIZIDE)

Sulphonylureas are first-line treatment in normal weight patients with type 2 diabetes (although some protocols suggest metformin as first line for all patients, irrespective of weight). They act by stimulating secretion of insulin from functioning pancreatic beta-cells. Sulphonylureas are considered in patients who are not overweight or in whom metformin is contraindicated or not tolerated. These drugs should be avoided if the patent has severe hepatic or renal impairment.[14] Sulphonylurea therapy satisfactorily controls glycaemia in about two-thirds of people with type 2 diabetes. Hyperinsulinaemia can occur, and may lead to hypoglycaemia and weight gain. If hypoglycaemia occurs, the dose should be reduced.

ALPHA GLUCOSIDASE INHIBITORS (E.G. ACARBOSE)

These drugs delay glucose absorption from the intestine, so reducing postprandial glucose levels and are an add-on treatment. They may provoke flatulence, diarrhoea or abdominal bloating so should be avoided in someone with irritable bowel.

PRANDIAL GLUCOSE REGULATORS (E.G. REPAGLINIDE, NATEGLINIDE)

These drugs increase the secretion of insulin by pancreatic beta-cells as sulphonylureas do, but the effects of these drugs depend on glucose levels because of the way their action is mediated.

GLITAZONES

These relatively new drugs act on the nuclear receptors in adipose tissue, termed the perixisome proliferator-activated receptors. Glitazones target the gamma-receptors to influence lipid and glucose metabolism, glucose transport and storage. They also reduce atherogenesis by direct effects on the vascular wall and coagulation. Glitazones can postpone insulin therapy for those with type 2 diabetes, by preventing the decline in pancreatic beta-cell function and preserving endogenous insulin secretion. Liver function tests should be measured before treatment is started then every two months for a year and periodically thereafter.[14]

COMBINATION THERAPY

As beta-cell function deteriorates and the circulating insulin levels are unable to overcome underlying tissue resistance, there is progressive loss of glycaemic control. The majority of patients with type 2 diabetes will require combination therapy to maintain adequate glycaemic control with an HbA_{1c} in the lower range, e.g. metformin and a sulphonylurea.

Glitazones should only be used in combination with metformin or sulphonylurea for patients who are unable to take either one of those drugs because of intolerance or a contraindication. That is, metformin and sulphonylurea combination therapy should remain the first choice where monotherapy has not produced adequate glycaemic control. Glitazones are not currently licensed in the UK for triple therapy in combination with those two drugs.[15]

INSULIN

Insulin should be considered for type 2 patients who are not adequately controlled by diet and/or oral hypoglycaemic agents alone or in combination. Insulin can be used in combination therapy with oral hypoglycaemic drugs such as sulphonylureas and biguanides. For instance, in an overweight patient, metformin may be continued simultaneously with insulin up to 850 mg three times daily (but many prescribers limit the dose to 1 gm twice daily).

Usually the decision to introduce insulin has been negotiated with people with type 2 diabetes, over a considerable time. The patient should understand the reasons why their blood glucose control is worse and the pros and cons of insulin. They will have probably have contributed to their management by self-monitoring of blood sugars. This phase of diabetes care can be very demanding and often involves the help of experts from outside the practice with a special interest and expertise in diabetes. Patients should be reviewed frequently until their blood glucose control and HbA$_{1c}$ have stabilised.

ANTIHYPERTENSIVE TREATMENT

Research supports a target diastolic pressure of no more than 80 mmHg in people with diabetes to reduce the risk of major cardiovascular events.[5] ACE inhibitors, diuretics, beta-blocking drugs and calcium channel blockers all reduce cardiovascular morbidity and mortality. The reduction in blood pressure, rather than the particular drug used, seems to matter most. Many patients with type 2 diabetes need a combination of antihypertensive agents to maintain low blood pressures. Around a third of subjects included in the United Kingdom Prospective Diabetes Study (UKPDS) trial required three or more antihypertensive treatments to achieve effective blood pressure control.[16]

STATINS

There is important research to support *all* people with type 2 diabetes taking statins, irrespective of their age, sex, baseline levels of total or LDL cholesterol or the presence of prior vascular disease.[5,17] There is no consensus yet as to whether all patients with types 1 and 2 diabetes should receive lipid-lowering drugs.[18]

Complications of diabetes

Macrovascular and microvascular complications are largely irreversible. Adults with diabetes are twice as likely to die each year as people without diabetes. Their life expectancy is reduced by an average of five to ten years.[19] A person with type 2 diabetes is two to four times more likely to suffer from heart disease, stroke and peripheral vascular disease than someone without diabetes.

Macrovascular complications of diabetes include cardiovascular disease, cerebrovascular disease and peripheral vascular disease. Stroke or circulatory problems of the lower limbs result in ischaemic pain, ulceration, gangrene and amputation.

Coronary heart disease death rates are several times higher in people with diabetes than in those without. Cardiovascular disease kills up to 75% of people with type 2 diabetes. The risk of coronary heart disease in people with diabetes cannot be explained by the presence of the classic risk factors for coronary heart disease – smoking, hypertension and raised serum lipid concentrations – diabetes seems to confer its own risk.[7]

Microvascular complications lead to retinopathy, nephropathy and neuropathy that occur alone or in combination with each other.

The longer a person has diabetes, the more likely they are to develop complications. Co-existing risk factors such as hypertension, hypercholesterolaemia and smoking cigarettes interact with diabetes to make complications more likely.

Table 8.1 describes the relative risks of various complications occurring in people with diabetes compared with people without diabetes.

Table 8.1:   Risks of morbidity associated with all types of diabetes mellitus[19]

Complication	Relative risk[a]
Blindness	20
End stage renal disease	25
Amputation	40
Myocardial infarction	2–5
Stroke 2–3	

[a]magnitude of risk compared with people without diabetes

Mortality and morbidity from diabetes is higher in people from lower socio-economic groups, the unemployed and in those who left full-time education at a young age.

The UKPDS trial showed that intensive control of blood glucose and tight control of blood pressure reduced the risk of microvascular complications.[20] The findings from the study are summarised in Box 8.1 below. Tight glycaemic control was classified as HbA_{1c} levels of 7.0% or less. Tight blood pressure control may be easier to achieve than tight glycaemic control for some individual patients, have fewer side-effects and make more of an impact on survival.

Any reduction in HbA_{1c} levels is likely to reduce the risk of complications. Each 1% reduction in mean HbA_{1c} levels was associated with 21% reduction in deaths related to diabetes.[21]

Box 8.1:   Summary of the United Kingdom Prospective Diabetes Study (UKPDS)[7,20]

- The UKPDS was a multicentre randomised controlled trial carried out in the UK that started in 1977.
- 4209 patients aged 25–65 years with newly diagnosed type 2 diabetes were randomly allocated to different therapies: 'conventional' diet and exercise therapy, or 'intensive' diet and exercise and oral hypoglycaemic or insulin therapy.
- Over the 10 years of the study, the mean HbA_{1c} in the intensively treated group was lower than that in the conventionally treated group (7.0% vs. 7.9% HbA_{1c}).
- The risk for any diabetes-related endpoint in the 'intensive' group was 12% lower than in the 'conventional' group.

- There was a 25% reduction in the risk of the microvascular endpoints between the two groups from 11.4 events to 8.6 events per 1000 patient years.
- There was no significant difference in any of the diabetes-related endpoints between therapy with chlorpropamide, glibenclamide or insulin.
- The lower mean blood pressure in the tight blood pressure control group of 144/82 mmHg compared with 154/87 mmHg was translated into lower risks of serious complications: 32% fewer deaths, 44% fewer strokes and 37% less microvascular endpoint damage.
- Most subjects randomised to the blood pressure control groups needed more than one antihypertensive treatment to effectively control their blood pressure.

The UKPDS trial demonstrated the association between raised lipids and death rates – from cardiovascular disease, heart attack, stroke, peripheral vascular disease, hypo- and hyperglycaemia and sudden deaths. Every reduction of 1 mmol/l in total cholesterol was associated with a 24% reduction in diabetes-related deaths over the 10.4 years' average follow up of the study. A 1 mmol/l decrease in LDL-cholesterol cut diabetes-related deaths by 25% and a 0.1 mmol/l increase in HDL-cholesterol was associated with a 7% reduction in diabetes-related deaths.[20]

Type 1 diabetes mellitus

Diagnosis of type 1 diabetes is usually straightforward if there are one or more symptoms of thirst, polyuria, malaise and weight loss, taken together with a raised blood glucose level and ketones in the urine (*see* page 160).

Case study 8.2

When Mr Wells comes for his diabetes review, you congratulate him on his current HbA_{1c} of 7.1% and fasting cholesterol of 3.9 mmol/l. His weight is steady and he has given up smoking cigarettes since you last saw him six months ago. He found it hard to stop as he had smoked for the last 10 years since he was 14 years old, and most of his friends still smoke. Even developing diabetes at the age of 16 years had not stopped him smoking, and it had taken a new girlfriend who objected to him smelling of cigarettes to help him quit. He has no microalbuminuria, and his blood pressure is 110/75 mmHg. Mr Wells has taken a statin daily for the last 12 months and his cholesterol level has fallen by 20%. He finds his pen injection device, which holds the insulin in cartridge form, simple and convenient to use. He has had several episodes of mild hypoglycaemia in the last six months, but on every occasion he knew that he had delayed eating for too long.

What issues you should cover

There is a great deal of evidence about the beneficial effects of improved blood glucose control on preventing and slowing the development of complications in type 1 diabetes.[5,7] Just as for type 2 diabetes, the better the glycaemic control the more effective is primary and secondary prevention of vascular, retinal, renal and neurological complications. The risk of developing microvascular complications is substantially reduced if people with type 1 diabetes achieve an HbA_{1c} of below 7.5%, according to the findings of the Diabetes Control and Complications Trial (DCCT) described in Box 8.2.

Box 8.2:   Summary of the Diabetes Control and Complications Trial (DCCT)[22]

- A randomised controlled trial carried out in the USA from 1986.
- 1441 patients with type 1 diabetes were randomly allocated to either 'intensive insulin therapy' (IIT) or conventional therapy.
- 99% of people with diabetes completed the study (except those that died).
- The results showed that IIT delays the onset and slows the progression of diabetic retinopathy, nephropathy and neuropathy.
- Any improvement in the control of diabetes prevents complications: the better the control, the fewer the complications.
- IIT increased the risk of severe hypoglycaemia occurring by three times.
- The results were so convincing that the trial was terminated after an average of 6.5 years.

Management of hypoglycaemic episodes

Hypoglycaemic episodes may be mild and easily reversed by the patient, severe requiring help from someone nearby, or profound resulting in coma or convulsions. The tighter the glycaemic control, the more likely the patient is to have a hypoglycaemic attack (or 'hypo'). A typical attack consists of pallor, sweating, shaking, hunger, light-headedness, tingling, slurred speech and confusion.

People with diabetes should carry dextrose or some other form of carbohydrate (glucose tablets or drink) with them at all times to take when they experience the warning signs of hypoglycaemia, to be followed by a snack or meal. Carers or relatives should be educated to watch out for signs of a hypo attack and intercede if the patient does not take action. A relative or carer can administer glucose gel (such as Hypostop) or 1 mg of glucagon subcutaneously or intramuscularly to treat a hypo if the dextrose or other carbohydrate has not worked. An intravenous load of 50 ml of 20% glucose (or 25 ml of 50% glucose) must be given by a clinician 10 minutes later if there is no response to the glucagon. People with diabetes should carry a card or bracelet describing their diagnosis and the treatment they take.

The frequency and severity of hypoglycaemic episodes can be minimised by adjusting insulin type, dosage and frequency and ensuring that meals or snacks are well timed. Short-acting insulin analogues such as lispro are absorbed faster and lead to improved post-prandial blood glucose levels. Another new alternative is insulin glargine that functions as a very long-acting insulin without peaks and troughs.[23]

Those on insulin should receive frequent instruction and reminders on injection technique and looking after their insulin and syringes. Discuss with them their blood glucose and ketone testing and what the results mean and when, why and how to deal with hypoglycaemia.

Insulin injection

Patients should be taught the basic injection technique, the rotation of injection sites, and information about mixing insulins in the syringe – soluble (clear) with a longer-acting (cloudy) insulin.

Patients with type 2 diabetes may be able to be managed on once a day intermediate-acting insulin or a mixture of short- and medium-acting insulin. This may be in addition to oral hypoglycaemic agents, particularly for elderly patients, for whom twice daily injections may not be feasible.

A twice-a-day short- and medium-acting mixture is popular for patients, injected before breakfast and before the evening meal. The ratio of short- and medium-acting insulin can be varied to suit lifestyle, work and also residual endogenous insulin production. These will vary over time and need frequent reappraisal. Fixed mixtures of soluble and isophane insulins are available in a range of proportions.

A 'basal-bolus' regime can give patients more flexibility. A short-acting insulin is given with food and an intermediate-acting insulin (usually isophane) is given before bedtime to cover overnight insulin requirements. This approach does offer greater flexibility but not necessarily better glycaemic control. It does suit people with unpredictable lifestyles and mealtimes – like Mr Wells in our case study. Pen devices are popular to administer the insulin, since they are portable and simple to use. There is a version suitable for the visually impaired. There is an upper limit of 70 units in the insulin cartridges, which varies between pen devices.

Insulin pump therapy or continuous subcutaneous insulin infusion can be given via a syringe worn underneath the patient's clothing. An adjustable basal infusion rate provides background insulin, supplemented by pre-meal insulin boluses administered by the patient. Such pumps have to be purchased by the patient.

If sugars are consistently high (rather than simply raised in response to a self-limiting viral illness for example), increase the dose of short-acting insulin by two units at a time up to 20% of the total insulin dose until the blood glucose control is improved.

The usage of metformin alongside insulin has increased for patients with type 1 diabetes, as for those with type 2, especially in those who are overweight, are receiving large doses of insulin, or have an HbA_{1c} above 8%.[23]

Education and psychological support for patients with diabetes

People with diabetes will benefit if they are well informed about their condition and able to participate in making decisions about the management of their condition. Good information will help people with diabetes make choices about their diet, smoking, physical activity and other health-related behaviour. Research has shown that self-management approaches are effective in increasing the use of beneficial behaviours, especially monitoring. But we have no real evidence of improvements in HbA_{1c} levels from such patient education initiatives (yet).[5,24] One project (the Dose Adjustment for Normal Eating (DAFNE) programme) involves an intensive five-day course that teaches patients to adjust their insulin requirements in accordance with their carbohydrate intake. The programme has been shown to produce improvements in blood glucose control and a reduction in HbA_{1c} of 1% over the subsequent six months.[11,25]

Individuals with type 2 diabetes may mistakenly believe that their condition is trivial because they are asymptomatic when they are first identified as having diabetes. You need to motivate them to comply with advice and treatment.

Your aim for people with diabetes is to enable them to take ownership of controlling their diabetes. They need to control blood glucose levels consistently, and reduce other risk factors as far as possible to achieve the ultimate goal of preventing acute and late complications of diabetes.[11]

The ultimate goal of patient education is to improve:

*   control of vascular risk factors – blood glucose levels, blood lipids and blood pressure
*   management of diabetes-associated complications
*   quality of life.

You may join others in advocating the 'expert patient' programme for patients living with long-term medical conditions including diabetes. Patients who have been through the programme themselves then lead the sessions and act as tutors for other patients. The programme covers individuals' confidence in accessing services, knowing how to act upon symptoms, dealing with acute attacks or exacerbations of their disease, making the most effective use of medication and treatment, and understanding the implications of the advice from health professionals.[1,11,26]

As a minimum for patient education, give patients simple written information leaflets (if they are literate) about diabetes, dietary advice etc and the contact details of Diabetes UK.[6]

Quality indicators in diabetes mellitus

There are 99 points available for diabetes mellitus in the GMS contract for general practice.[27] Collate the information from whenever patients are seen in primary or secondary care settings. There may be a mismatch between the annual quality indicators of the GMS contract and criteria specified in local and national guidelines; for instance for microalbuminuria testing and the lower levels of lipids and blood pressure recommended as best practice by various recent research studies.[12,17] The indicators are summarised in Table 8.2.

Table 8.2: Quality indicators in diabetes mellitus

Indicator		Points	Maximum threshold (%)
DM1	The practice can produce a register of all patients with diabetes mellitus.	6	
DM2	Percentage of patients with diabetes whose notes record BMI in the previous 15 months.	3	90
DM3	Percentage of patients with diabetes in whom there is a record of smoking status in the previous 15 months, except those who have never smoked where smoking status should be recorded once.	3	90
DM4	Percentage of patients with diabetes who smoke and whose notes contain a record that smoking cessation advice has been offered in the last 15 months.	5	90
DM5	Percentage of diabetic patients who have a record of HbA_{1c} or equivalent in the previous 15 months.	3	90
DM6	Percentage of patients with diabetes in whom the last HbA_{1c} is 7.4 or less (or equivalent test/reference range depending on local laboratory) in last 15 months.	16	50

DM7	Percentage of patients with diabetes in whom the last HbA_{1c} is 10 or less (or equivalent test/reference range depending on local laboratory) in last 15 months.	11	85
DM8	Percentage of patients with diabetes who have a record of retinal screening in the previous 15 months.	5	90
DM9	Percentage of patients with diabetes with a record of the presence or absence of peripheral pulses in the previous 15 months.	3	90
DM10	Percentage of patients with diabetes with a record of neuropathy testing in the previous 15 months.	3	90
DM11	Percentage of patients with diabetes who have a record of their blood pressure in the past 15 months.	3	90
DM12	Percentage of patients with diabetes in whom the last blood pressure is 145/85 mmHg or less.	17	55
DM13	Percentage of patients with diabetes who have a record of microalbuminuria testing in the previous 15 months (except patients with proteinuria).	3	90
DM14	Percentage of patients with diabetes who have a record of serum creatinine testing in the previous 15 months.	3	90
DM15	Percentage of patients with diabetes with proteinuria or microalbuminuria who are treated with ACE inhibitors (or A2 antagonists).	3	70
DM16	Percentage of patients with diabetes who have a record of total cholesterol in the previous 15 months.	3	90
DM17	Percentage of patients with diabetes whose last measured total cholesterol within previous 15 months is 5 or less.	6	60
DM18	Percentage of patients with diabetes who have had influenza immunisation in the preceding 1 September to 31 March.	3	85

All minimum thresholds are 25%

Collecting data to demonstrate your learning, competence, performance and standards of service delivery

Example cycle of evidence 8.1

- Focus: clinical care
- Other relevant foci: repeat prescribing; preconception care

Stages of the evidence cycle

Stage 1
Select targets

Stage 2
Set standards

Stage 5
Document it all

Stage 3A/B
Identify needs

Stage 4
Learning/action plan

Case study 8.3

Miss Hope comes to see you to renew her three-monthly contraceptive injection and tells you casually that this may be her last injection as she and her partner are hoping to try for a baby later in the year. Your interest is immediately engaged as Miss Hope has type 1 diabetes. Your nurse practitioner leads on diabetes for your practice team, and you refer Miss Hope to him (yes we mean him!) for a review of her diabetes control and preparation for conception and pregnancy. He reminds you that local guidelines specify that you should refer all patients with type 1 diabetes who are planning a pregnancy to a specialist in secondary care.

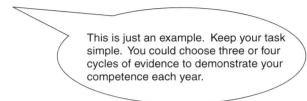

This is just an example. Keep your task simple. You could choose three or four cycles of evidence to demonstrate your competence each year.

Stage 1: Select your aspirations for good practice

The excellent GP:

- has the knowledge and skills to optimise the health and wellbeing of pregnant patients as part of their routine care
- can provide best practice in chronic disease care (including diabetes) whether or not they have a particular responsibility for that clinical area within the primary care team
- knows when to share the care of patients with specialists in primary or secondary care.

Stage 2: Set the standards for your outcomes

Outcomes might include:

- the way learning is applied
- a learnt skill
- a protocol
- a strategy that is implemented
- meeting recommended standards.

- Know and apply best practice in the care of women with diabetes who anticipate becoming, or are, pregnant.
- The practice protocol for shared care of pregnant women with diabetes is agreed by community midwives, GPs, practice nurses and diabetes experts in secondary care.

Stage 3A: Identify your learning needs

- Self-assess your knowledge and skills about managing diabetes care proactively for women who are pregnant or are contemplating pregnancy.
- Review your reflective log. Reflections may identify areas where you are unsure of what best practice is, for preconception care or management of diabetes.

- Obtain feedback from the nurse practitioner who is leading on diabetes care in your practice team as to his perceptions and observations about your knowledge and practice when he sees your patients for follow-up.

Stage 3B: Identify your service needs

Any of the needs assessment exercises in 3A may also reveal service needs.

- Audit the diabetic control in women with diabetes at their first antenatal consultation and at intervals thereafter (HbA_{1c}, fasting blood glucose, blood glucose at other times of day).
- Arrange an ongoing audit of outcomes of pregnancy for patients with diabetes. This might be undertaken as a significant event audit for a case of premature labour, or birth of an infant with low/excessive weight or other adverse outcome. Or it might be an audit across the PCO that you tap into, so that there are sufficient numbers to make the audit work.
- Join a working group in the PCO that is reviewing service planning of Standard 9 in the Diabetes NSF for England or the equivalents in Scotland, Wales and Northern Ireland.[1] Be part of the group reviewing, implementing and auditing local protocols for the management of pregnant women with diabetes. Compare your results from your own practice with what is expected.

Stage 4: Make and carry out a learning and action plan

- Attend a workshop on best practice in the care of those with diabetes.
- Shadow or sit in with an expert in diabetes to observe the management of patients who are pregnant, e.g. a hospital consultant or a practitioner with a special interest in diabetes.
- Take a module about diabetes by undertaking a distance learning programme.
- Attend a working party or represent your practice or PCO that is composing or updating its clinical care protocol in relation to diabetes or maternity care.
- Run an in-house educational session to introduce and discuss the application of a practice-based clinical care protocol.

Stage 5: Document your learning, competence, performance and standards of service delivery

- Keep a copy of the local audit protocol developed to address Standard 9 of the Diabetes NSF.[1]

- Audit records from the practice, e.g. a significant event audit and the subsequent action plan.
- Include the current practice-based protocol for shared care of patients with diabetes, including those who are pregnant.
- Include your reflective notes from your log book, or from shadowing an expert in diabetes, or from feedback on your practice from colleagues.
- Include your certificate of completion of the distance learning module and/or workshop.

Case study 8.3 continued

Your nurse practitioner arranges for Miss Hope to meet with the nurse consultant with a specialism in diabetes to review and improve her diabetic control. Miss Hope also revisits the dietitian to discuss her current diet and how that might change once she is pregnant. Miss Hope is booked in with your nurse practitioner for a smoking cessation session as she usually smokes 5–10 cigarettes a day.

Example cycle of evidence 8.2

- Focus: relationships with patients
- Other relevant foci: clinical care; education of patients; teamwork

---

Case study 8.4

You decide as a practice team to try and improve the knowledge and skills of patients with diabetes (both types 1 and 2) that you care for, in the self-management of their condition. You want to help patients change their lifestyles as far as possible.

> This is just an example. Keep your task simple. You could choose three or four cycles of evidence to demonstrate your competence each year.

Stage 1: Select your aspirations for good practice

The excellent GP:

- supports patients in taking control of the management of their disease as far as possible
- motivates their patients to adopt a healthy lifestyle.

Stage 2: Set the standards for your outcomes

Outcomes might include:

- the way learning is applied
- a learnt skill
- a protocol
- a strategy that is implemented
- meeting recommended standards.

- A structured education programme is available to patients with diabetes.
- Patients with diabetes who have participated in the structured education programme have increased knowledge about the course of diabetes, its treatment and the prevention of complications.

Stage 3A: Identify your learning needs

- Ask the next 10 consecutive patients with diabetes who consult you which type of diabetes they have, what risks they run from having diabetes and how they and health professionals can reduce the risks of diabetes. Reflect on the extent to which your patients appear to need education about their condition.

- Explain to a doctor or nurse with special expertise or interest in diabetes your plan for how you might educate your patients about their condition. Ask for their views on your intended approach and how likely it is to have an impact on patients.

Stage 3B: Identify your service needs

> Any of the needs assessment exercises in 3A may also reveal service needs.

- Find out what structured education programmes for patients with diabetes already exist in your locality or are planned.
- Undertake a baseline audit in your practice of HbA_{1c} as a marker of blood glucose control for all patients with diabetes reviewed in the previous year. Assess what proportion have an HbA_{1c} under 7.5%, and discuss as a team what justification there is for establishing a structured education programme for patients with diabetes.

Stage 4: Make and carry out a learning and action plan

- Contact Diabetes UK for information about patient education programmes.[6]
- Read up on how others have established patient education programmes and discuss with GPs and nurses in your practice team or locality.[11,25, 26, 28]
- Attend a health promotion workshop on 'How to motivate patients' with your practice nurse who leads on diabetes care in your practice.
- Invite the local nurse with a special interest in diabetes to attend a working group meeting in your practice to discuss setting up a patient education programme.

Stage 5: Document your learning, competence, performance and standards of service delivery

- Include your plan for a structured education programme for patients with diabetes who are registered with your practice.
- Audit the HbA_{1c} levels of patients attending the programme, before starting and at the next annual diabetes check.
- Keep your notes from the literature and correspondence with Diabetes UK, and your discussions with local experts.
- Include your certificate of attendance at the health promotion workshop.

Case study 8.4 continued

You set up a series of six educational sessions for patients with diabetes in the early evening. These are held once a month and run by you and the practice nurse with a lead in diabetes. Thirty-one patients attend in all, of whom 25 attend all sessions relevant to their type of diabetes, some of whom also bring relatives or carers. The local diabetes nurse with a special interest in diabetes talks at two of the sessions, explaining about converting to insulin in type 2 diabetes, and minimising the risk of complications of diabetes. You have yet to undertake the subsequent annual reviews to find out whether the HbA_{1c} levels of those patients who attended the sessions have shown an improvement.

Example cycle of evidence 8.3

- Focus: good medical practice
- Other relevant focus: adherence to protocol for chronic disease management

Stages of the evidence cycle

Stage 1
Select targets

Stage 2
Set standards

Stage 5
Document it all

Stage 3A/B
Identify needs

Stage 4
Learning/action plan

Case study 8.5

Mr Payne has come to consult you about his back pain. After taking a history and examining him, you ask why he has not returned before now about his diabetes – as it eight months since you diagnosed him with type 2 diabetes and advised him to start a healthy diet and lose weight, before being considered for antidiabetic medication. It is obvious from his reply that he did not understand that he should attend before his annual review. Your GP partner who is the diabetes lead is on a three-month sabbatical and the practice nurse who runs the diabetic clinic is leaving at the end of the week and you are in the midst of appointing her successor. So you must sort Mr Payne out and are unsure of the details of the practice protocol for newly diagnosed diabetes.

This is just an example. Keep your task simple. You could choose three or four cycles of evidence to demonstrate your competence each year.

Stage 1: Select your aspirations for good practice
The excellent GP:

- has a reasonable basic knowledge about the management of common chronic diseases, whether or not they have lead responsibility in the practice for a clinical condition.
- adheres to an agreed practice protocol describing the accepted approach to the management of a chronic disease.

Stage 2: Set the standards for your outcomes

Outcomes might include:

- the way learning is applied
- a learnt skill
- a protocol
- a strategy that is implemented
- meeting recommended standards.

- Adhere consistently to the protocol for the practice management of patients with diabetes.

Stage 3A: Identify your learning needs

- Undertake a significant event audit as to why Mr Payne's care lapsed and he did not return to monitor his blood glucose control and start further treatment. Talk the situation through with Mr Payne to find out why your initial instructions about follow-up care were misconstrued.
- Ask the practice nurse who has run the diabetes review clinic to comment on the standards of your care of people with diabetes before she leaves her post.
- Self-assess your knowledge of the practice protocol on diabetes.

Stage 3B: Identify your service needs

> Any of the needs assessment exercises in 3A may also reveal service needs.

- As a practice team, review the register of diabetes and check in ensuing consultations with all the practice team that all patients with confirmed diabetes are entered on the register.
- Run an audit to check the percentage of patients on the register who have a record of: BMI, smoking status, HBA_{1c}, cholesterol and serum creatinine, retinal screening, testing for peripheral pulses and neuropathy, blood pressure, a check for microalbuminuria and influenza vaccination – in the last 15 months.
- Compare the practice protocol for the management of diabetes with the quality indicators that are part of the GMS contract to check that it is synchronous.[27]

Stage 4: Make and carry out a learning and action plan

- Brush up on any gaps in your knowledge of best practice in the management of diabetes, over and above the requirements of the quality outcomes framework of the GMS contract[27] by reading up on the NSF, NICE guidelines and the evidence (look at the references at the end of this chapter).
- Attend a seminar to update yourself on diabetes management run by the multidisciplinary diabetes specialist team in a protected learning time session organised by your PCO.
- Organise an in-house educational session when your GP colleague returns from sabbatical and the new practice nurse is appointed. Agree everyone's roles and responsibilities in everyday surgeries and the diabetic review clinic in line with the agreed practice protocol on the management of diabetes.

Stage 5: Document your learning, competence, performance and standards of service delivery

- Include a copy of the revised practice protocol, specifying the responsibilities and roles of team members.
- Record the results of six-monthly re-audits of the proportion of patients achieving the indicators in the quality outcomes framework.
- Keep notes on the significant event audit of Mr Payne's delayed follow-up and subsequent action to minimise recurrence, e.g. a patient information sheet is prepared for patients newly diagnosed with diabetes, including a description of how the practice operates diabetes care.
- Retain your certificate of attendance at the protected learning time session.

Case study 8.5 continued

Mr Payne's next HbA_{1c} is 8.0% and you start him on metformin, building up the dose gradually, in accordance with the practice protocol. He understands the importance of returning for regular follow-up. The new practice nurse already has a university diploma in diabetes management and soon establishes fail-safe systems for looking after patients with diabetes.

References

1   NHS Executive (2001) *National Service Framework for Diabetes.* Department of Health, London.

2   Chambers R, Stead J and Wakley G (2001) *Diabetes Matters in Primary Care.* Radcliffe Medical Press, Oxford.

3   Scottish Intercollegiate Guidelines Network (1996) *Management of Diabetes in Pregnancy. National Clinical Guideline for Scotland.* Scottish Intercollegiate Guidelines Network, Edinburgh.

4   World Health Organization (1999) *Definition, Diagnosis and Classification of Diabetes Mellitus and its Complications – Part 1: diagnosis and classification of diabetes mellitus.* World Health Organization, Geneva.

5   Godlee F (ed.) (2004) *Clinical Evidence.* Issue 11. BMJ Publishing Group, London.

6   Diabetes UK (1997) *Recommendations for the Management of Diabetes in Primary Care.* Diabetes UK, London. www.diabetes.org.uk

7   Williams R and Farrar H (2001) Diabetes mellitus. In: *Health Needs Assessment Series; the epidemiologically based needs assessment reviews.* Radcliffe Medical Press, Oxford.

8   King's Fund Policy Institute (1996) *Counting the Cost: the real impact of non-insulin-dependent diabetes.* King's Fund, London.

9   Smith S (2003) Newly diagnosed type 2 diabetes mellitus. 10-minute consultation. *British Medical Journal.* **326:** 1371.

10 Albert KG (1992) Good control or a happy life? In: I Lewin and C Seymour (1992) *Current Themes in Diabetes Care.* Royal College of Physicians, London.

11 National Institute for Clinical Excellence (2003) *Guidance on the Use of Patient-education Models for Diabetes.* Technology Appraisal Guidance 60. National Institute for Clinical Excellence, London.

12 Williams B, Poulter NR, Brown M *et al.* (2004) British Hypertension Society guidelines for hypertension management 2004 (BHS-IV): summary. *British Medical Journal.* **328:** 634–40.

13 National Institute for Clinical Excellence (2004) *Type 2 Diabetes. Prevention and management of foot problems.* Clinical Guideline 10. National Institute for Clinical Excellence, London.

14 Joint Formulary Committee (2004) *British National Formulary. BNF 47.* British Medical Association and the Royal Pharmaceutical Society of Great Britain, London.

15 National Institute for Clinical Excellence (2003) *Glitazones for the Treatment of Type 2 Diabetes.* Technology Appraisal Guidance 63. National Institute for Clinical Excellence, London.

16 UK Prospective Diabetes Study Group (1998) Tight blood pressure control and risk of macrovascular and microvascular complications in type 2 diabetes: UKPDS 38. *British Medical Journal.* **317:** 703–12.

17 Heart Protection Study Collaborative Group (2002) MRC/BHF Heart Protection Study of cholesterol lowering with simvastatin in 20 536 high-risk individuals: a randomised placebo-controlled trial. *Lancet.* **360:** 7–22.

18 National Institute for Clinical Excellence (2002) *Management of Type 2 Diabetes. Management of Blood Pressure and Blood Lipids.* Inherited Clinical Guideline H. Reference no 167. National Institute for Clinical Excellence, London.

19 Scottish Intercollegiate Guidelines Network (1997) *Management of Diabetic Cardiovascular Disease. National Clinical Guideline for Scotland.* Scottish Intercollegiate Guidelines Network, Edinburgh.

20 United Kingdom Prospective Diabetes Study (UKPDS) Group (1998) Intensive blood-glucose control with sulphonylureas or insulin compared with conventional treatment and risk of complications in patients with Type 2 diabetes (UKPDS 33). *Lancet.* **352:** 837–53.

21 Stratton IM, Adler AI, Neil AW *et al.* (UKPDS Group) (2000) Association of glycaemia with macrovascular and microvascular complications of type 2 diabetes (UKPDS 35): prospective observational study. *British Medical Journal.* **321:** 405–12.

22 Diabetes Control and Complications Trial (DCCT) Research Group (1993) The effect of intensive treatment of diabetes on the development and progression of long-term complications in insulin-dependent diabetes mellitus. *New England Journal of Medicine*. **329:** 977–86.

23 Devendra D, Liu E and Eisenbarth GS (2004) Type 1 diabetes: recent developments. *British Medical Journal*. **328:** 750–4.

24 Coster S, Gulliford MC, Seed PT *et al.* (2000) Monitoring blood glucose control in diabetes mellitus: a systematic review. *Health Technology Assessment*. **4 (12)**.

25 Gadsby R (2003) Promoting self-management in diabetes. *The Practitioner*. **247:** 318–21.

26 Department of Health (2001) *The Expert Patient: a new approach to chronic disease management in the 21st century*. Department of Health, London.

27 General Practitioners Committee/The NHS Confederation (2003) *New GMS Contract. Investing in general practice*. General Practitioners Committee/NHS Confederation, London.

28 Audit Commission in Wales (2003) *Diabetes Services in Wales*. Audit Commission, London.

9

Thyroid disease

Hypothyroidism

Case study 9.1

When you first saw Mrs Weary last week she had consulted you because she had felt 'tired all the time' for the last six months. On questioning, she admitted that she had gained a stone in weight in the last year but had not eaten any more than usual. She felt a bit down but attributed that to her nearing 60 years of age. She has come back to hear the results of blood tests you organised last week. Her blood count, renal and liver function and fasting glucose are normal. Her TSH level is raised at 6.6 mu/l and her thyroxine level is normal at 17.4 pmol/l. You diagnose her as having subclinical hypothyroidism.

What issues you should cover

Like Mrs Weary, up to 10% of women over 60 years of age have subclinical hypothyroidism with moderately raised TSH and normal free thyroxine (T_4) levels.[1] Most people in this category do not progress to overt hypothyroidism. The advice is to simply observe the thyroid function over time (e.g. with annual testing of TSH) without treating their subclinical state with thyroxine.[2] Research is inconclusive about the benefits of treating subclinical hypothyroidism; such treatment can induce hyperthyroidism and reduce bone mass in post-menopausal women and increase the risk of atrial fibrillation, as for overt hypothyroidism.[1] A consensus statement by the American Association of Clinical Endocrinologists and the Royal College of Physicians recommends that levothyroxine therapy is appropriate in patients with a TSH over 10 mu/l, who are the most likely to progress from subclinical to overt hypothyroidism.[2]

Hypothyroidism occurs in around 4 in 1000 women on average, rising to 8 in 1000 people over 70 years old. Women are six times more likely to suffer from hypothyroidism than men. The symptoms and signs are generally a more extreme version of those described by Mrs Weary, with gradual onset of symptoms, increasing lethargy and depression, memory loss and intolerance of the cold. Other symptoms include hair loss, puffy eyes, husky voice, bradycardia, constipation, dizziness, irregular menstruation, infertility, dementia, and delayed relaxation of tendon reflexes.[1,3] With primary hypothyroidism (myxoedema) the thyroid gland may not be palpable and be atrophic, or the patient may have the firm, irregular goitre of Hashimoto's thyroiditis. Primary hypothyroidism occurs after destruction of the thyroid gland because of an autoimmune state (i.e. chronic autoimmune thyroiditis) or medical intervention such as surgery, radioiodine or radiation treatment or the side-effects from drugs such as amiodarone or lithium. Secondary hypothyroidism occurs after damage to the pituitary gland or hypothalamus.[1]

Levothyroxine is the treatment of choice for maintenance treatment for overt hypothyroidism, usually at a dose between 100 and 200 µg daily, which can be administered as a single dose.[4] The aim is to achieve a serum TSH within the normal range. Overtreatment is indicated by a raised free T_4 and suppressed TSH, and is associated with such adverse consequences as an increased risk of developing atrial fibrillation and death from vascular disease, and reduced bone mineral density in postmenopausal women.

Hyperthyroidism

Case study 9.2

Mrs Race thought that her hot sweats were due to the menopause at first but her periods were still regular. Although she was only 40 years old she knew that it came early in some women. But then she started losing weight even though she had a voracious appetite. Her husband who accompanies her to see you says she is irritable and difficult to live with nowadays – she cannot sit still and relax with him in the evenings. She is not the same woman he had married five years previously.

She volunteers that her heart seems to be racing at times, and she feels more tired than usual. She wonders if her thyroid might be playing up as her mother takes tablets for an underactive thyroid. Examining her you find a medium-sized, firm goitre that is mobile as you palpate it. There is no lymphadenopathy. Mrs Race has a fast, regular pulse of about 96 beats per minute. Her palms are sweaty and she has a fine tremor of both hands when her arms are out-stretched. Her eyes appear normal – no sign of lid retraction or lid lag or exopthalmus. Subsequent blood tests show a normal full blood count and confirm thyrotoxicosis with low TSH and raised free thyroxine (T_4) and free tri-iodothyronine (T_3) levels. You do not check her female hormone levels.

What issues you should cover

Thyrotoxicosis is 10 times more common in women than men. About 1–2% of women in the UK develop thyrotoxicosis. In most, their thyrotoxicosis is due to an autoimmune disorder such as Graves' disease. Mrs Race's symptoms and signs are a typical presentation with thyrotoxicosis.[3]

The extent to which you initiate treatment before Mrs Race is seen by a specialist in thyroid disease will depend on local arrangements and waiting times to be seen in secondary care. All patients with a new diagnosis of hyperthyroidism should be referred to a specialist when they present, for a cause to be defined and treatment plan established.[2] If there is a delay, you as the GP will confirm the biochemical diagnosis of thyrotoxicosis and check the full blood count noting a normal white count, and then initiate treatment with e.g. 30–40 mg of carbimazole for 4–8 weeks until the patient is euthyroid. After that you will titrate the dose against the patient's TSH levels and probably reduce the dose of carbimazole to 5–15 mg for the next 12–18 months, in collaboration with the hospital specialist. Propanolol may be used as an adjunct to treatment for those patients such as Mrs Race with a tremor or tachycardia who need symptom relief – for example 10–40 mg propanolol 3–4 times per day or nadolol 80–160 mg per day.[4] Beta-blockers may also be used in preoperative preparation for thyroidectomy as it renders the thyroid gland less vascular, thus making surgery easier.

The specialist assessment will distinguish different causes of hyperthyroidism such as Graves' disease, toxic-nodular hyperthyroidism and thyroiditis.

Case study 9.2 continued

The specialist confirms that Mrs Race has Graves' disease. Mrs Race develops a rash over her trunk which is very itchy, but these side-effects lessen with your prescription for a long-acting antihistamine and she continues with her carbimazole therapy, stepping down her starter dose of 30 mg per day after 6 weeks to 15 mg per day. Twelve months later she is taking 5 mg per day and at 18 months she stops taking carbimazole. Five years later she is still attending for yearly monitoring of her T_4 and TSH levels which remain in the normal range.

Not everyone has such a straightforward course as Mrs Race. If rash and pruritus triggered by carbimazole do not settle, the patient may be switched to propylthiouracil. The serious complication of agranulocytosis occurs in 0.3% of patients treated with antithyroid drugs. The Committee on Safety of Medicines warns that all patients starting carbimazole should be advised to report any signs of infection such as sore throat immediately. A white blood cell count should be undertaken if there is any clinical sign of infection. Carbimazole should be stopped immediately if there is any clinical or laboratory evidence of neutropenia.[4]

Radioactive iodine is used increasingly for the treatment of thyrotoxicosis in all age groups, particularly when compliance with taking carbimazole is a problem, or in patients with co-existing problems such as cardiac disease, or after relapse of the thyrotoxicosis such as after thyroidectomy.[4] Early radioiodine is increasingly selected as the treatment of choice. The small radiation dose to the gonads from a therapeutic dose of radioiodine has been likened to that from an intravenous pyelogram and presents a minimal or no risk to future fertility. Radioiodine is contraindicated in pregnancy or breast feeding, and pregnancy should be avoided for 4–6 months after treatment.

Indications for thyroid surgery – a subtotal thyroidectomy – depend on the patient's symptoms and preferences for surgery over alternative treatments. Where there is obstruction from a toxic multinodular goitre, surgery may be the treatment of choice. Patients are treated with antithyroid drugs for three months before surgery to render them euthyroid for the operation. This is to avoid surgery (or similarly, radioiodine therapy) precipitating a thyrotoxic crisis.

Patients who are treated with radioiodine or have thyroid surgery should be placed on a practice disease register and have their thyroid function tested annually. Fifty per cent will become hypothyroid over time and require prescribed levothyroxine. There is a 50% relapse rate after stopping carbimazole, so annual follow up should continue indefinitely for these patients too. They should then be considered for radioiodine or thyroid surgery.

Thyroid cancer

Case study 9.3

Mrs Globe looks worried as she asks you to look at the lump in her neck. This is one of her rare visits – in all of her 70 years she has seldom consulted a doctor. It is a few weeks since she has noticed the lump and as she has no other symptoms she has put off coming to you. You examine the lump, noting if it is part of the thyroid or other part of the neck, if it moves on swallowing and if cervical lymph nodes are palpable. You arrange blood tests for thyroid function but consider the most likely diagnosis to be thyroid cancer.

What issues you should cover

Thyroid cancer is rare, accounting for about 1% of all cancers. The overall 10-year survival rate for differentiated thyroid cancer is about 80–90%. Between 5% and 20% of patients with thyroid cancer develop local or regional recurrences and 10–15% develop distant metastases.[5]

The presence of associated symptoms or signs indicate advanced disease. Look for hoarseness which may arise from vocal cord palsy, cervical lymphadenopathy, stridor resulting from airway obstruction, or distant bone pain indicating spread of the cancer.

Refer a solitary thyroid nodule urgently to a surgeon or endocrinologist specialising in thyroid cancer, to be seen within two weeks of referral if you suspect it is a cancerous thyroid lump. At the same time, check thyroid function to investigate the possibility of hyperthyroidism or hypothyroidism associated with thyroid goitre.[4] If the results are normal and the patient is euthyroid, that makes the diagnosis of thyroid cancer more likely. A malignancy is more likely if the patient is male, aged under 20 years or over 60 years, has a short history, has a history of radiation or has lymphadenopathy.

If the diagnosis is confirmed as cancer by a fine needle aspiration, the patient will normally undergo a total thyroidectomy. Any remaining thyroid tissue will then be treated with radioactive iodine. Cancers that do not take up radioiodine are treated with radiotherapy. Levothyroxine replacement therapy is used to suppress TSH levels (<0.1 mu/l). Thyroglobulin is monitored thereafter as a marker of residual or recurrent thyroid tumour. A thyroid cancer specialist multidisciplinary team should provide follow-up to ensure early detection of any recurrence or complications.[5]

Quality indicators in thyroid disease[6]

Table 9.1:   Quality indicators in thyroid disease

Indicator		Points	Maximum threshold (%)
Thyroid 1	The practice can produce a register of patients with hypothyroidism.	2	
Thyroid 2	The percentage of patients with hypothyroidism with thyroid function tests recorded in the previous 15 months.	6	90

All minimum thresholds are 25%

Cases of thyroid cancer would feature within the requirement for practices to produce a register of all cancer patients as part of the quality and outcomes framework, and be reviewed within six months of confirmed diagnosis – to include an assessment of support needs, if any, and a review of the co-ordination arrangements with secondary care.

Collecting data to demonstrate your learning, competence, performance and standards of service delivery

Example cycle of evidence 9.1

- Focus: clinical care
- Other relevant focus of evidence: repeat prescribing

Stages of the evidence cycle

Stage 1 – Select targets

Stage 2 – Set standards

Stage 3A/B – Identify needs

Stage 4 – Learning/action plan

Stage 5 – Document it all

Case study 9.4

Flicking through a prescribing journal, you read an article about the drug amiodarone and wonder if all of the patients on this drug in your practice are being monitored as they should be.[4] You are particularly concerned to read about the true story of a 79-year-old woman who had a fall as a result of hypothyroidism induced by amiodarone where the patient's thyroid function was not monitored.[7]

This is just an example. Keep your task simple. You could choose three or four cycles of evidence to demonstrate your competence each year.

Stage 1: Select your aspirations for good practice

The excellent GP:

- arranges long-term monitoring of prescribed drugs that have potentially serious side-effects
- understands the side-effects of drugs she/he prescribes.

Stage 2: Set the standards for your outcomes

Outcomes might include:

- the way learning is applied
- a learnt skill
- a protocol
- a strategy that is implemented
- meeting recommended standards.

- An audit of the practice protocol for monitoring long-term use of amiodarone shows that all patients prescribed this drug have their thyroid and liver function tested every six months.

Stage 3A: Identify your learning needs

- Read the article about amiodarone in the medical press and consider if you already know and understand the content.[7]
- Keep a reflective log and note down any educational needs arising from the prescription of amiodarone as patients present for follow-up care, or as you read hospital letters describing the initiation of treatment.
- Discuss the possible initiation of amiodarone by GPs with an expert on prescribing, e.g. the prescribing adviser for the PCO, to find out if there is anything that you do not know.

Stage 3B: Identify your service needs

> Any of the needs assessment exercises in 3A may also reveal service needs.

- Undertake an audit of the extent to which all patients in the practice who receive repeat prescriptions for amiodarone have had their thyroid function checked in the last six months.
- Undertake a significant event audit of at least one case identified above where a patient on amiodarone has not had thyroid function checked in the previous 12 months. Identify the reasons for the lack of monitoring.
- Check whether GPs or nurse prescribers are over-ruling alerts triggered by the computer system when certain drugs are prescribed together, without considering the alert seriously. Discuss with colleagues in an open and non-judgemental way to find out.

Stage 4: Make and carry out a learning and action plan

- Read up about amiodarone. Look at the indications, the likelihood of thyroid dysfunction, the monitoring required to watch for hypothyroidism, the risks of pneumonitis, hepatotoxicity, etc. Check that you know about possible drug interactions with cimetidine, digoxin, warfarin, phenytoin, beta-blockers and other drugs.
- Learn to undertake a search using the practice computer to select patients taking repeat prescriptions of particular drugs and ascertain how many have had monitoring blood tests performed within certain timescales. Arrange a tutorial from the practice expert or the computer software suppliers. Then delegate the task on a regular basis to a reliable staff member who has dedicated time for such monitoring and has the responsibility specified in his/her revised job description.

Stage 5: Document your learning, competence, performance and standards of service delivery

- Record the results of the audit of the practice protocol on the prescribing of amiodarone, and the associated six-monthly monitoring of thyroid and liver function together with the findings from your action plan.
- Include the job description of the staff member whose role is to undertake monitoring of repeat prescriptions as directed by the GP.

Case study 9.4 continued

All patients who are being prescribed amiodarone have had their thyroid function tested before the drug was initiated, but only 50% have had their thyroid function tested in the previous year. You write to invite those who have not had their thyroid function checked in the previous six months to make an appointment for their blood tests. One month later, only one patient's test is still outstanding, and you are reassured to find that all the patients had normal thyroid function (normal T_4, T_3 and TSH levels).

Example cycle of evidence 9.2

- Focus: good medical practice
- Other relevant foci: relationships with patients; informed choice

Stages of the evidence cycle

Stage 1
Select targets

Stage 2
Set standards

Stage 5
Document it all

Stage 3A/B
Identify needs

Stage 4
Learning/action plan

Case study 9.5

Mrs Rush has just had a miscarriage at 12 weeks. She has two children already, and developed thyrotoxicosis when the second child was one year old. Since then her thyrotoxicosis has been controlled with carbimazole – one year later she is taking 10 mg carbimazole per day and her TSH is within normal levels. She has come to see you to discuss the possibility that the carbimazole caused the miscarriage and to discuss alternative options for treatment. She is especially keen to consider thyroid surgery so that she will not have to take drugs any more.

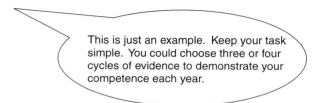

This is just an example. Keep your task simple. You could choose three or four cycles of evidence to demonstrate your competence each year.

Stage 1: Select your aspirations for good practice

The excellent GP:

- understands the various alternative options for treatment of a disease
- can explain alternative options for treatment to a patient so that they can make an informed choice.

Stage 2: Set the standards for your outcomes

Outcomes might include:

- the way learning is applied
- a learnt skill
- a protocol
- a strategy that is implemented
- meeting recommended standards.

- Up-to-date literature and recommendations for internet sites relevant to the treatment of thyroid disease are available to patients in the practice.
- Patients are able to make an informed choice about treatment options, having discussed their management and any concerns with you at their consultation.

Stage 3A: Identify your learning needs

- Self-assess whether you know about possible teratogenic effects of carbimazole or other drugs prescribed for thyroid disease (e.g. propylthiouracil, beta-blockers), or radioiodine.
- Discuss Mrs Rush with a group of GP colleagues (e.g. at a trainers' workshop) and practise explaining the pros and cons of treatment options for thyrotoxicosis – medication, radioiodine and thyroidectomy. Ask colleagues for feedback about the content of your talk and the way in which you conveyed the options – were you confident, did you explain in a way that would easily

be understood by patients? Alternatively, ask the patient for feedback after the real consultation – explaining that you are trying to improve your consulting style. You could audiotape your real consultation with the patient's permission and critique your own performance afterwards, or ask a colleague to comment.

Stage 3B: Identify your service needs

> Any of the needs assessment exercises in 3A may also reveal service needs.

- Find out what treatment options the local thyroid specialist provides and his/her preferences for the alternative regimens of antithyroid drugs, thyroidectomy and radioiodine. Do this by letter, phone call or an arranged or opportunistic face-to-face meeting.
- Request copies of information given to patients by the thyroid specialist team in secondary care. Check whether you understand the content and be ready to explain any medical terms or jargon to patients.

Stage 4: Make and carry out a learning and action plan

- Make the most of your learning from any of the needs assessment exercises in Stages 3A and 3B. Make notes of the points to emphasise or the changes you want to put into practice.
- Prepare an up-to-date information file for patients with hyperthyroidism and hypothyroidism, including simple explanations of their disease or condition, warnings, alternative approaches to treatment, importance of monitoring for the rest of their lives, useful (and dependable) websites. Draw much of this material from what you already have in the practice, from dependable texts[1,2,4] and what you obtained from the multidisciplinary specialist thyroid team in hospital.

Stage 5: Document your learning, competence, performance and standards of service delivery

- Include a copy of the patient information file for hyperthyroidism and hypothyroidism.
- Make notes on the feedback on your consultation style, explaining alternative approaches in relation to hyperthyroidism and your subsequent reflections.

Case study 9.5 continued

Mrs Rush listens carefully to your explanation about the possible options for treating hyperthyroidism and the benefits and risks of taking carbimazole, in particular the advice on taking it during pregnancy and breast feeding. As she is interested you look at the advice in the *British National Formulary*[4] together – and she decides to continue with carbimazole. You are able to reduce the dose still further to 5 mg per day and you arrange to recheck her thyroid function soon after.

Example cycle of evidence 9.3

- Focus: clinical care
- Other relevant foci: practice management; record keeping

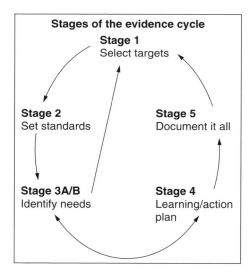

Stages of the evidence cycle

Stage 1
Select targets

Stage 2
Set standards

Stage 5
Document it all

Stage 3A/B
Identify needs

Stage 4
Learning/action plan

Case study 9.6

Your colleagues have nominated you to be the clinical lead for thyroid disease in your practice. This is not really as grand as it sounds. They mean that you should be able to answer everyone's queries about best practice in managing thyroid disease, ensure that the practice is gaining the maximum quality points for managing thyroid disease, and know how to manage any patients with complicated problems that involve thyroid disease.

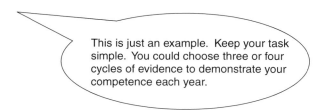

This is just an example. Keep your task simple. You could choose three or four cycles of evidence to demonstrate your competence each year.

Stage 1: Select your aspirations for good practice

The excellent GP:

- consistently applies best practice in their management of patients' chronic conditions
- generates maximum quality points for the practice while working to high standards of patient care
- provides guidance for colleagues who have less expertise than they do, in particular clinical fields.

Stage 2: Set the standards for your outcomes

Outcomes might include:

- the way learning is applied
- a learnt skill
- a protocol
- a strategy that is implemented
- meeting recommended standards.

- All patients with confirmed hypothyroidism are entered on the register for this group, and no patient is on the disease register in whom hypo-thyroidism has not been confirmed by thyroid function tests.[6]
- All patients with hypothyroidism on that disease register have had at least one thyroid function test recorded in the previous 15 months.[6]

Stage 3A: Identify your learning needs

- Write down a description of your responsibilities as clinical lead for thyroid disease in the practice and check with colleagues that your understanding coincides with theirs.
- Sit in with a consultant specialist in thyroid disorders for two outpatient clinic sessions, to check that your knowledge of best practice is up to date,

and identify areas of practice or management with which you were previously unfamiliar.

Stage 3B: Identify your service needs

> Any of the needs assessment exercises in 3A may also reveal service needs.

- Arrange for a member of the practice staff to undertake an audit under your direction. Audit whether all patients with confirmed hypothyroidism are entered on the register, and no patient is on the disease register in whom hypothyroidism has not been confirmed with thyroid function tests. Search under 'thyroxine' and 'levothyroxine', then check each patient's record to confirm the diagnosis. Add the approved Read code unless already entered.
- Arrange for an audit to monitor that all patients with hypothyroidism on that disease register have had at least one thyroid function test recorded in the previous 15 months. Ensure both electronic and manually entered results have the correct Read code.

Stage 4: Make and carry out a learning and action plan

- Make the most of sitting in with the consultant specialist to learn more about thyroid disease and options for management, as well as to identify your learning needs.
- Check your knowledge of approved Read codes and make up a practice directory of codes for all disease areas linked to quality points.[6]
- Read up on best practice of the management of thyroid disorders.[1,2,4]

Stage 5: Document your learning, competence, performance and standards of service delivery

- Keep copies of the results of the audits that can be submitted to justify your quality points.
- Keep a list of your responsibilities as the clinical lead for thyroid disease for your appraisal portfolio.
- Include your list of approved Read codes in connection with quality points.
- Keep notes summarising the learning points and detailing your gaps in knowledge and skills to inform the next revision of your PDP.

Case study 9.6 continued

Everyone is pleased with you when the practice achieves maximum points for the register of patients with hypothyroidism as nearly all the patients with hypothyroidism have had thyroid function tests recorded in the previous 15 months.

References

1 Nygaard B (2004) Primary hypothyroidism. In: F Godlee *Clinical Evidence*. **Issue 11:** 807–12. BMJ Publishing Group, London.

2 Vanderpump MP, Ahlquist JAO, Franklyn J *et al.* (1996) Consensus statement for good practice and audit measures in the management of hypothyroidism and hyperthyroidism. The Research Unit of the Royal College of Physicians, the Endocrinology and Diabetes Committee of the Royal College of Physicians and the Society for Endocrinology. *British Medical Journal.* **313:** 539–44.

3 Souhami RL and Moxham J (eds) (2002) *Textbook of Medicine.* Churchill Livingstone, London.

4 Joint Formulary Committee (2004) *British National Formulary. BNF 47.* British Medical Association and the Royal Pharmaceutical Society of Great Britain, London.

5 British Thyroid Association and Royal College of Physicians (2002) *Guidelines for the Management of Thyroid Cancer in Adults.* Royal College of Physicians, London. www.rcplondon.ac.uk

6 General Practitioners Committee/The NHS Confederation (2003) *New GMS Contract. Investing in general practice.* General Practitioners Committee/NHS Confederation, London.

7 Neil K (2004) Drug interactions: amiodarone and thyroid dysfunction. *Prescriber.* **19 March:** 62–4.

10

Dermatology

This chapter is not a complete guide to the management of the many dermatological conditions that a GP is likely to see. Rather, it gives the GP a model of how to gather evidence to demonstrate clinical competence in the management of patients with dermatological conditions.

Eczema

Case study 10.1

Peter Prickle is five years old. His mother has noticed a red itchy rash particularly in the popliteal and antecubital fossae. She has been treating this with a moisturising lotion, but this appears to have 'stopped working'. On examination his skin is generally dry. The areas of concern are erythematous with a poorly defined edge and evidence of excoriation. The distribution of the rash is approximately symmetrical. You note a slight yellow crusting in the left antecubital fossa.

Issues you should cover for eczema and any chronic skin condition

Similar principles may be applied when dealing with any chronic skin condition. The diagnosis should be given to the patient (and, where applicable, the patient's carer). Discuss with the patient/carer their understanding of the diagnosis you have given. Reinforce any information as necessary, and correct any misconceptions regarding the condition. You should aim to arrive at a mutually agreed model of the condition that is in line with current understanding of the condition's pathogenesis. You will then be able to provide the patient with a rationale for the options for treatments available.

Share information and discuss possible treatments with the patient. Explain how the particular treatment fits into the model of the disease process given. Describe the risks and intended benefits of different treatments. You should arrive at a final treatment regime for the patient's condition by mutual agreement, the patient having a clear understanding of the role, relative risks and intended benefits of each treatment element. Taking time to explain all aspects to the patient (and carer as appropriate) should improve concordance.[1]

In Peter's case, the dermatological diagnosis is eczema. This is a chronic inflammatory process typified by erythema, dry, slightly scaly skin, itch and a tendency to secondary infection. The crusting in the left antecubital fossa is consistent with a secondary infection with *Staphylococcus aureus*.

Case study 10.1 continued
You explain to Peter Prickle and his mother that the rash is eczema. You ask Mrs Prickle if she knows much about eczema. She tells you that she has heard of it, but states that she has no particular knowledge.

Following the outline of issues to be covered as given above, you devote the rest of the consultation to working through the following areas:

- sharing information with the patient (patient education) – knowledge
- agreeing treatment
- sharing information with the patient (patient education) – skills
- agreeing follow up
- health promotion
- patient/parent empowerment.

Patient education: knowledge

Concordance is arguably the soundest basis on which any condition may be optimally managed.[1] To achieve good concordance both doctor and patient (and/or the patient's carer) must share an agreed common understanding of the aetiology, pathogenesis, pharmacological and non-pharmacological treatment of the condition. So agree a working model of atopic eczema with Mrs Prickle.

A commonly used model of eczema is:

- the skin is a barrier, keeping substances inside the body in and substances outside the body out
- in eczema the skin becomes inflamed and this barrier function is lost

- irritants from outside can travel through the outer layer of the skin worsening this inflammation and so further compromising the barrier function
- certain substances can dramatically worsen inflammation. The most noted of these is the bacteria, *Staphylococcus aureus*. Unfortunately *Staphylococcus aureus* often colonises eczematous skin. A sudden flare-up of eczema may therefore be triggered by infection with *Staphylococcus aureus*.

The principles of treatment are therefore to:

1 *improve the skin's ability to act as a barrier* by:
   - not removing natural oils: avoid soaps, use soap substitutes instead e.g. aqueous cream
   - supplementing the effect of natural oils by using emollients, both on the skin and added to the bath
   these measures will form the mainstay of treatment
2 *suppress inflammation*. This is achieved with topical corticosteroids. An alternative approach is to use an immunomodulatory agent such as topical tacrolimus or picrolimus
3 *treat staphylococcal infection*. Options include anti-staphylococcal additives present in some emollients, topical antibiotics and systemic antibiotics.

Case study 10.1 continued

You discuss the information as above with Mrs Prickle. She feels happy with the model and explanation used. She expresses reservations regarding the use of steroids on Peter as she has heard that steroids can cause severe side-effects. Why else would they be banned from people taking part in sport?

Agree treatment

The intended benefits as well as the cautions and side-effects of each treatment should be discussed with the patient and/or their carer. This allows them to make an informed choice as to whether or not a specific treatment is acceptable.

Mrs Prickle seems willing to accept a regime of soap avoidance and use of emollients for her son. There are many possible combinations. In general these consist of an emollient applied between two and four times daily (the more the better), a soap substitute e.g. aqueous cream or emulsifying ointment, and a bath additive e.g. balneum or oilatum.

If there still seems to be a lack of shared understanding regarding the nature of topical corticosteroids, clarify the risks and benefits.

Case study 10.1 continued

Having discussed the cautions regarding an emollient regime, particularly the fact that the bath additive will make the bath really slippery, Mrs Prickle agrees that emollients are an acceptable treatment. You then go on to discuss corticosteroid treatment for Peter. You explain the difference between corticosteroids and the anabolic steroids that are occasionally abused by athletes. You acknowledge Mrs Prickle's concerns regarding the potential of steroids to cause side-effects. You spend some time discussing these, including thinning of the skin, striae formation and the potential for suppression of the adreno-cortico axis in overuse of potent topical corticosteroids. You also explain that sparing usage of topical corticosteroids with the least potent steroid that will control the eczema is the key principle of treatment. Mrs Prickle tells you that this approach now makes sense and she is agreeable to the sparing use of the milder topical corticosteroids if it is necessary. By agreement you therefore prescribe 1% hydrocortisone cream to be applied twice daily as directed.

As there is clinical evidence of staphylococcal infection, you suggest a five-day course of oral flucloxacillin. Mrs Prickle concurs. You have now arrived at an agreed treatment regime.

If Mrs Prickle had refused treatment with steroids, at least you would have done your best to ensure that such a refusal would be an informed decision.

Patient education: skills

It is important that the patient and/or their carer understand how to use the treatments given. Box 10.1 gives information about the prescribing of appropriate quantities of topical treatment in eczema.

Box 10.1:   Prescribing appropriate quantities of topical treatment in eczema

Topical steroids

The amount of topical corticosteroid required for any given period is calculated from the amount of fingertip units (FTUs) required to treat the area, multiplied by the number of treatments per day (usually two), multiplied by the number of days' treatment. This divided by two gives the required quantity of steroid cream in grams. That is:

the number of FTUs required for treatment × number of treatments per day × number of days treatment required ÷ 2 = amount of steroid cream required in grams.

The approximate amounts required for twice daily applications for an adult are given in table form in the *British National Formulary*.[2]

Emollients

Often insufficient quantities are prescribed. To cover both arms in an adult twice a day for one week will require between 100 g and 200 g of cream or ointment or 200 ml of lotion. Approximate quantities required for twice weekly application to specific areas of an adult for one week are given in the *British National Formulary*.[2,3]

In the current case study of Peter, a five-year-old boy with eczema, the following information will apply:

- emollients should be applied liberally, in the direction of hair fall
- topical corticosteroids should be applied sparingly, usually twice daily
- a commonly used method to ensure correct application of corticosteroid creams is the fingertip unit. One fingertip unit is the amount of cream squeezed from the tube onto the volar aspect of the index finger from the crease overlying the distal interphalangeal joint to the tip of the finger. This approximates to 0.5 g of cream. This amount is sufficient to cover a surface area equivalent to the palmar surface of both hands.
- a patient leaflet will help reinforce correct usage.

Case study 10.1 continued

You explain how to apply the emollients and the topical corticosteroid creams to Mrs Prickle, reinforcing the demonstration and information with explanatory leaflets.

Agree follow-up

The course of Peter's eczema will be variable. He may grow out of it; or it may persist into adulthood. It is likely that he will experience flares and remissions. So, follow-up needs to be arranged with medical staff or nursing staff. The interval between follow-ups will depend on the severity of the eczema and on the preferences and attitudes expressed by the patient or, in this case, his mother.

Health promotion

The presence of eczema implies that the skin will be more likely to react to irritants in later life. Even at Peter's age you can discourage a career choice that will involve skin contact with irritants, such as being a motor mechanic, hairdresser or nurse. Although not specifically related to a diagnosis of eczema, sun avoidance is another important dermatological area of health promotion.

Avoid overloading Mrs Prickle with information too early. It may be better if these messages are left until the patient is followed up.

Patient (or carer) empowerment

Eczema is a chronic disease. Whether Peter grows out of his eczema or whether it persists into adulthood, it is important for the patient/patient's carer to feel able to manage the condition. Ideally a point should be reached where the doctor's role is that of an expert resource to utilise when problems arise. The day-to-day management of the condition should be the patient's/carer's domain.

As a doctor you therefore need to encourage the development of appropriate knowledge, skills and attitudes in the patient and his mother. This has been started already by following the process outlined above. Add resources in the form of information leaflets, books, web addresses and contact details of any patient support or self-help groups.

Case study 10.1 continued

You give Mrs Prickle a leaflet produced by the National Eczema Society. This includes their contact details.[4] You ask them if there are any points that require clarification. Mrs Prickle feels that she has understood what you have told her and the options for management.

Pigmented naevi

Case study 10.2

Audrey Blemish, a 45-year-old lady, presents to you because she has noticed a 'mole' on her head. She was watching a documentary about skin cancer on the television last night and is now extremely worried that this mole is a cancer.

Issues you should cover in any acute dermatological condition and any new or changing mole

It is possible to apply aspects of this case to any acute dermatological condition, including a new or changing mole.

The consultation will need to deal with the following areas:

- recognise the patient's concern
- arrive at a diagnosis. If diagnosis is unclear explain possible diagnoses: explain why it is necessary to reach a more definitive diagnosis and explain how this may be achieved:
    - if by biopsy discuss as for any minor surgical procedure
    - if by referral to secondary care explain intended benefits of this
    - if by other investigations discuss specificity and sensitivity of investigation
- ensure the patient understands the significance of the diagnosis as well as any degree of uncertainty relating to the diagnosis
- discuss treatment options with the patient:
    - be able to discuss advantages, disadvantages and effects on prognosis for each possible treatment path, including the option of no treatment
    - if the management of a condition requires skills or facilities not available in general practice, explain the advantages and disadvantages of proposed treatment
    - if you are uncertain how best to manage a condition, explain the need to obtain a more expert opinion and how this will be obtained. Options may include referral to secondary care or telephone advice from consultant
- reach agreement with the patient as to which treatment path is to be followed
- initiate treatment or referral
- arrange follow up as appropriate
- give health promotion advice (patient education for the long term).

All the above items will empower the patient by providing knowledge and skills that are not only applicable to the presenting complaint but are also transferable to similar conditions that may affect the patient in the future.

Ultimately it will be the patient who decides what they want to do. By following the above procedures that decision will at least be informed.

Recognise the patient's concern

In this case study the patient has been 'up front' with her concern. She wants to know whether or not she has a skin cancer. Specifically she wishes you to exclude malignant melanoma.

Arrive at a diagnosis

This will follow the standard medical pattern of history, examination and possibly investigations.

TAKE A HISTORY

In terms of background information:

- does she have a history of sunburn as a child?
- does she have a personal or family history of malignant melanoma?

Specifically you will want to know if this is a new mole or whether it has always been there. If the mole is longstanding has there been any changes in:

- size
- shape
- pigmentation?

Whether new or longstanding, has the mole been inflamed, oozed or bled? Has Mrs Blemish experienced any itch or altered sensation in the mole? If she has noticed any of these changes over what time period has this occurred?

MAKE AN EXAMINATION

You should examine for and document:

- the position of the mole
- the size of the mole
- the shape (regular or irregular) of the mole
- whether pigmentation is regular or irregular
- whether the mole is flat or raised. If raised is its profile regular or irregular?
- whether there are any signs of bleeding, oozing or inflammation.

A size over 6 mm, irregularity of shape and/or pigmentation and/or profile in a new mole or change in size or shape or pigmentation in a pre-existing mole should be regarded as suspicious. A history or signs of bleeding, oozing or inflammation should also be viewed as suspicious of malignancy.

Case study 10.2 continued

Mrs Blemish tells you that she thinks she has had the mole since her early teenage years. She is sure that it used to be flat. It seems to have become raised, although on thinking about it she feels that this change happened slowly some years ago. She does not believe that there have been any recent changes. She has no personal or family history of skin cancer. You examine the mole and find a 5 mm diameter, hemispherical papule with uniform light brown pigmentation situated on the left parietal aspect of her scalp. On inspection you note hairs growing from it.

The description given is consistent with a diagnosis of a benign intradermal melanocytic naevus. This will need no action unless the site of the naevus is troublesome, for example if it is catching on clothing.

Case study 10.2 continued

You explain that the mole has no features that cause concern and you therefore believe it to be benign. Mrs Blemish is relieved. She asks you if you are '100% certain' that the mole is and will always be benign?

DISCUSS DIAGNOSTIC CERTAINTY

It is impossible to give such a guarantee as a '100% certainty' as to its being benign. It is important that Mrs Blemish is aware of this. One approach you might take is to state that as far as can be seen there are no malignant features present (changes that a mole often exhibits if it is undergoing malignant change).

Moles can and should be monitored by the patient over their lifetime.

Discuss treatment options

The pros and cons of removing a benign-looking mole are presented in Box 10.2.

Box 10.2:   Pros and cons of minor surgical removal of a skin lesion

Benefits

- Skin lesion is removed – although in some instances it may recur
- Histological diagnosis is (usually) obtained

Disadvantages

- Pain – both with local anaesthetic and postoperatively
- The procedure *will* leave a scar

Risks

- Infection
- Recurrence of lesion (largely dependent on type of lesion and method of removal)
- Keloid scar formation, especially in sternal and deltoid areas of skin
- Damage to underlying structures – depending on the site

Case study 10.2 continued

Your advice would be to keep the mole under observation with a view to acting at once should any of these changes indicating possible malignancy occur. You explain that an alternative is to remove the mole. This *will* leave a scar. There is a risk of keloid scar formation. Should this occur it will be cosmetically less acceptable than retaining the original mole. You discuss the further risks and benefits of removal of the mole as detailed in Box 10.2. You also discuss the pros (avoid the cons of surgery) and cons (skin lesion still in skin, slightly less clarity regarding diagnosis) of not having the lesion removed.

Reach agreement with patient as to the treatment path to be followed

Mrs Blemish decides that she does not wish to have the mole removed. There is therefore no treatment to be initiated.

Arrange follow-up as appropriate

In the case study here, the most sensible follow-up is patient-led. It would consist of her monitoring the mole and initiating medical contact as and when problems occur.

Health promotion (patient education for the long term)

Health promotion advice is extremely important in this case study, as the education received will be central to triggering the patient-initiated follow-up discussed above.

There are two obvious aspects that revolve around this case:

- mole surveillance
- sun protection.

> **Case study 10.2 continued**
>
> You advise Mrs Blemish regarding 'mole surveillance', as detailed in Box 10.3. You explain to her that should she notice any of the changes detailed, she should return to her GP at once for further assessment. You also advise her regarding adopting sun protection of her skin as detailed in Box 10.4 and using sunscreens (*see* Box 10.5).
>
> You reinforce both messages with patient leaflets. Mrs Blemish say she has no further questions and leaves your surgery reassured.

Advise the patient to monitor all moles. Changes in a mole should prompt the patient to have it checked by a doctor. The features given in Box 10.3 are indicative of a possible malignant melanoma. The first three features are 'major features' and would almost always prompt further investigation. Any moles showing any of these features should be checked by the patient's GP, for the sake of the greatest patient safety.

> **Box 10.3:**   Mole surveillance to detect signs of malignancy
> * Change in size
> * Change in shape – especially if shape is irregular with a ragged outline
> * Change in colour – especially if colour is variegated shades of brown or black
> * Itch
> * Redness or inflammation
> * Bleeding, oozing or crusting

Ultraviolet (UV) light is harmful to the skin. It is associated with solar age changes, including loss of elasticity, wrinkles and solar elastosis. Sun and other UV exposure leads to actinic keratosis, increases the risk of squamous cell carcinoma of the skin, and basal cell carcinoma. They are also associated with the development of malignant melanoma. It therefore makes sense for people to systematically protect their skin from excessive sunlight – as detailed in Box 10.4.

> **Box 10.4:**   Adopting sun protection
> * Wear clothing such as long sleeved shirts and broad brimmed hats to give additional sun protection.
> * Remember that the sunlight will be stronger when on holiday nearer the equator.
> * Avoid being in the sun between 11am and 3pm when it is at its strongest.

- Apply a high protection factor sun block (e.g. SPF 25, 4 star or better, *see* Box 10.5) before going out.
- Re-apply sun block regularly and liberally.
- Shelter under a beach umbrella which will reduce sun exposure, but not prevent it altogether.
- Avoid sitting where the sun will be reflected onto you e.g. by white sand, white buildings or water.

Ultraviolet radiation is divided into three wave bands. These are ultraviolet A (UVA), ultraviolet B (UVB) and ultraviolet C (UVC). UVC is screened out by the atmosphere. Protection is therefore needed against UVA and UVB as detailed in Box 10.5.

Box 10.5:   Sunscreens, SPF and UV protection

Sunscreens work by either reflecting or absorbing ultraviolet light. Some do both. They have separate ratings for UVA (expressed as a star rating) and UVB (expressed as a SPF number).

UVB causes sunburn. Protection against this is tested by application of sunscreen to an area of skin and then exposing the skin to ultraviolet. The time taken for the skin to develop an erythematous reaction is compared with the time taken for the same reaction to occur in non-protected skin. This is expressed as a ratio to give the sun protection factor (SPF), e.g. skin protected with SPF 2 would take twice as long to burn as unprotected skin. The amounts of sunscreen per unit surface area used by patients in real life are usually significantly less than the amounts used when testing SPFs. It is therefore extremely unlikely that the degree of protection given in reality will be as high as the degree obtained in the testing laboratory.

The SPF test is based on a sunburn response and therefore can give no indication of protection against UVA. Sunscreens are given a star rating for UVA protection. The highest rating is four stars.

Quality indicators relating to patient experience

There are no specific indicators for dermatology in the quality and outcomes framework.[5] But many of the generic indicators about record keeping and good practice management apply to consultations about dermatology. For example, the information on quality points relating to patient experience given in Table 10.1 is just as relevant for patients with skin conditions as for other clinical fields.

Table 10.1: Quality indicators relating to patient experience

Indicator	Points
PE 1 Length of consultations The length of routine booked appointments with the doctors in the practice is not less than 10 minutes (if the practice routinely sees extras during booked surgeries, then the average booked consultation length should allow for the average number of extras seen in a surgery session. If the extras are seen at the end, then it is not necessary to make this adjustment). For practices with only an open surgery system, the average face-to-face time spent by the GP with the patient is at least 8 minutes. Practices that routinely operate a mixed economy of booked and open surgeries should report on both criteria.	30
PE 2 Patient surveys The practice will have undertaken an approved patient survey each year.	40
PE 3 Patient surveys The practice will have undertaken a patient survey each year, have reflected on the results and have proposed changes if appropriate.	15
PE 4 Patient surveys The practice will have undertaken a patient survey each year and discussed the results as a team and with either a patient group or Non-Executive Director of the PCO. Appropriate changes will have been proposed with some evidence that the changes have been enacted.	15

Collecting data to demonstrate your learning, competence, performance and standards of service delivery

Example cycle of evidence 10.1

- Focus: clinical care
- Other relevant foci: maintaining good medical practice; relationships with patients

Stages of the evidence cycle

Stage 1
Select targets

Stage 2
Set standards

Stage 5
Document it all

Stage 3A/B
Identify needs

Stage 4
Learning/action plan

Case study 10.3

Sarah Scratch is a 24-year-old woman who has recently joined your practice. This is the first time she has attended surgery other than to have a 'new patient' check with the practice nurse three weeks ago. She is concerned regarding her eczema, which seems to have recently flared up. She was using 'some creams from time to time'. These ran out about six weeks ago and she decided to see if she could manage without. She cannot remember which creams she used, but feels sure that one of them was a steroid cream. She tells you that she is not happy about steroids because of their side-effects. She has a friend who has heard of a new eczema treatment that does not involve steroids – she is keen to try this although she cannot remember the name of it.

This is just an example. Keep your task simple. You could choose three or four cycles of evidence to demonstrate your competence each year.

Stage 1: Select your aspirations for good practice

The excellent GP:

- maintains his or her knowledge and skills, and is aware of his or her limits of competence
- takes time to listen to patients and allow them to express their concerns
- uses clear language appropriate to the patient
- has a structured approach to long-term health problems and preventive care.

Stage 2: Set the standards for your outcomes

Outcomes might include:

- the way learning is applied
- a learnt skill
- a protocol
- a strategy that is implemented
- meeting recommended standards.

- Use consistent best practice in the management of eczema with good communication with patients.
- Have a consistent structured approach to the long-term management of eczema.

Stage 3A: Identify your learning needs

- Self-assess your confidence in diagnosing and managing eczema.
- Reflect on whether you are aware of new treatments for eczema.
- Perform a significant event audit of any cases where you feel that your management of eczema has been suboptimal. Discuss your findings with another colleague for their objective input about your performance.

- Survey the next 10 patients who consult with eczema. Establish how clearly they have understood your explanations of their condition at previous consultations and the nature and purpose of the treatments that you have prescribed.

Stage 3B: Identify your service needs

> Any of the needs assessment exercises in 3A may also reveal service needs.

- By distributing a short eczema knowledge quiz to team members, establish whether the advice given to patients from different members of the practice team is consistent,
- Locate all written patient information regarding the management of the eczema and review whether it is up to date and consistent with your practice protocol.
- Check whether information is available to patients at the practice regarding other sources of information such as from the National Eczema Society.
- Audit the last 10 patients seen with new diagnoses of eczema (by identifying the Read coding of conditions on practice computer). Establish how many have records of receiving written advice regarding:
  - the role of emollients in the management of eczema
  - correct steroid usage, including finger tip unit dosing of topical corticosteroids
  - contact details of the National Eczema Society.[4]

Stage 4: Make and carry out a learning and action plan

- Arrange a visit to sit in at a dermatology outpatient clinic, or community-based nurse-led eczema clinic. Visit one of these by yourself or take other relevant practice staff e.g. your practice nurse.
- Find or arrange a learning event covering the management of eczema. Learn about wet wraps, and appropriate use of topical tacrolimus and pimecrolimus.
- Formulate or update a practice guideline on the diagnosis and management of eczema. Discuss and agree it with others in the practice team.
- Produce or update a patient information leaflet on eczema. Ensure that this covers all the areas necessary to meet the standards that you have set out in your practice protocol.
- Review the explanation of eczema you give to your patients. Amend it as you feel appropriate.

Stage 5: Document your learning, competence, performance and standards of service delivery

- Document all of the above work undertaken in Stages 3 and 4.
- Keep your notes of the significant event audit action plan and achievements.
- Record the patient survey and conclusions.
- Keep a summary of the staff quiz and subsequent educational session.
- Include examples of relevant and current patient literature on eczema.
- Copy your diary entry relating to the session sitting in at the outpatient clinic.
- Include your reflections on the learning events attended and the evidence of putting learning into practice.

Case study 10.3 continued

Sarah Scratch has moderately severe flexural eczema with an area of impetigo at the left wrist. Listening to her ideas and concerns regarding her eczema and her expectations regarding treatment, you realise that:

- management of her eczema has been somewhat haphazard
- she did not see the reasoning behind aspects of her treatment and thus concordance has been low
- today's presentation has been precipitated by a flare-up of the eczema, probably triggered by infection with *Staphylococcus aureus*.

You explain your understanding of eczema to Ms Scratch in simple language and outline the 'model' of eczema. You explain the rationale behind the treatment of eczema with both emollients and topical corticosteroids, and recommend a short course of topical and systemic antibiotics.

You present the results of a patient survey on the management of eczema at a practice meeting. As your survey shows there are inconsistencies in eczema management, you arrange an educational meeting for all clinical staff at the practice, and a local dermatology consultant. A practice-based guideline on eczema management is agreed and includes the newer treatments and when to refer to the community-based dermatology nurse service for wet wraps.

Four weeks later, Ms Scratch's eczema is much better controlled. You discuss alternative treatments, but as her eczema has improved you reduce the potency of Ms Scratch's topical corticosteroid to the milder hydrocortisone. She continues to use emollients.

Some months later your practice receives a 'thank you' card from Sarah Scratch. You pin it up on the staff notice board.

Example cycle of evidence 10.2

- Focus: working with colleagues
- Other relevant foci: clinical care; communication

Stages of the evidence cycle

Stage 1
Select targets

Stage 2
Set standards

Stage 5
Document it all

Stage 3A/B
Identify needs

Stage 4
Learning/action
plan

Case study 10.4

Arthur Naevus is a 72-year-old man. His wife has noticed a pigmented area on Mr Naevus' back and brings him to your surgery. She thinks that this might have changed in size and colour. On examination you find a lesion overlying the left scapula. It is 1 cm in diameter, irregular in outline and irregularly pigmented. You tell Mr Naevus and his wife that this lesion has some suspicious features and you will refer him to a consultant dermatologist.

This is just an example. Keep your task simple. You could choose three or four cycles of evidence to demonstrate your competence each year.

Stage 1: Select your aspirations for good practice

The excellent GP:

- makes appropriate judgements about patients who need referral
- accompanies referrals with the information needed by the specialist to make an appropriate and efficient evaluation of the patient's problem
- maintains his or her knowledge and skills, and is aware of his or her limits of competence
- takes time to listen to patients and allow them to express their concerns
- uses clear language appropriate to the patient.

Stage 2: Set the standards for your outcomes

Outcomes might include:

- the way learning is applied
- a learnt skill
- a protocol
- a strategy that is implemented
- meeting recommended standards.

- Use consistent best practice in the management of pigmented lesions.
- Adopt appropriate referral patterns for skin lesions that raise suspicions of malignancy.
- Consistently include such information with referrals as to enable appropriate and efficient evaluation of the patients' problems.

Stage 3A: Identify your learning needs

- Establish what information is needed for 'appropriate and efficient evaluation' of pigmented lesions from good practice guidance (*see* Box 10.3 and previous text in this chapter).
- Reflect on your confidence in differentiating between benign and malignant pigmented naevi.
- Audit the histological diagnosis of any pigmented lesions you have sent off or cases you have referred urgently to secondary care as being possibly malignant in e.g. the last two years. Establish what percentage proved to be benign.
- Carry out a significant event audit on any cases where lesions you initially thought to be benign eventually proved to be malignant. Discuss your findings with another colleague to gain their insights about your practice.

Stage 3B: Identify your service needs

> Any of the needs assessment exercises in 3A may also reveal service needs.

- Review the practice system that ensures that all suspected malignant melanomas are referred under the 14-day 'possible cancer' system. Audit referrals made to ensure that this system exists and works effectively.
- Review the advice concerning pigmented lesions given to patients from different members of the practice team by patient survey (e.g. by direct questionnaire to patients by post or telephone).
- Check whether the practice provides patients with any written information regarding the warning signs to watch for in pigmented naevi.
- Discuss as practice team whether the practice as a whole promotes sun protection and capture, then make action plan to address gaps and learning lessons.
- Collect all written advice available to patients about pigmented naevi and sun protection. Check that it is all up to date and discard outdated literature.
- Audit the last 10 patients who consulted you to express concern regarding pigmented naevi and who did not require referral. Are there records of how many received written advice regarding sun protection and warning signs?
- Audit referral letters for the information contained. Are these letters of a satisfactory standard?

Stage 4: Make and carry out a learning and action plan

- Arrange a visit to a dermatology outpatient clinic. While there ask what information the consultant would like in a referral letter, to give the best clinical picture of the patient being referred.
- Find or arrange a learning event covering the management of pigmented naevi.
- As a practice team, discuss the results of the audits undertaken to identify learning and service needs. Learn from each other and share best practice.
- Use your learning time to formulate or update your practice guideline on the diagnosis and management of pigmented naevi.
- Produce or update a patient leaflet on pigmented naevi and sun protection. Ensure that this covers all the areas necessary to meet the standards you have set in Stage 2.

Stage 5: Document your learning, competence, performance and standards of service delivery

- Include a copy of your good practice guidance.
- Keep records of your audits of histological diagnosis, appropriate contents of referral letters and accuracy of dermatological referrals.
- Include your notes of the significant event audit plus the subsequent action plan.
- Include the summary of the patient survey with the patients' details anonymised.
- Keep notes of the action planning at practice meetings relating to ways of promoting sun protection.
- Include copies of patient literature relating to pigmented naevi, sun protection or other relevant topics.

Case study 10.4 continued

You refer Mr Naevus urgently under the 14-day suspected cancer rule. His lesion is excised. Histology confirms a malignant melanoma. Fortunately, as this was acted on promptly the Breslow thickness reported is 0.8 mm, giving a 93% chance of a five-year survival rate.[3] Some weeks later he attends the surgery to thank you for being such a good doctor and referring him urgently.

Example cycle of evidence 10.3

- Focus: relationships with patients
- Other relevant focus: maintaining trust

Case study 10.5

Melanie Mole presents in surgery with two lesions she wishes to have removed. The first is a 6 mm non-pigmented pedunculated papule, overlying the left lateral aspect of the thorax. She says that this has started to catch on her clothing and is therefore painful. The second lesion is a 5 mm flat uniformly pigmented naevus on the tip of her left shoulder. She asks if this can be removed at the same time. Both lesions have remained unchanged for many years. On examination you are convinced that both lesions are benign. You consider the ramifications of agreeing to Ms Mole's request.

This is just an example. Keep your task simple. You could choose three or four cycles of evidence to demonstrate your competence each year.

Stage 1: Select your aspirations for good practice

The excellent GP:

- gives patients information they need about their problem in a way that they can understand
- involves patients in decisions about their care
- obtains informed consent to treatment.

Stage 2: Set the standards for your outcomes

> Outcomes might include:
>
> - the way learning is applied
> - a learnt skill
> - a protocol
> - a strategy that is implemented
> - meeting recommended standards.

- Patients are given the information they need about their problem in a way that they can understand. (In this case this will include potential benefits of surgery, risks and potential complications of surgery and any risks arising from not performing surgery.)
- Patients are involved in decisions about their care.
- Informed consent is obtained in all cases where minor surgery is performed.

Stage 3A: Identify your learning needs

- Reflect on your knowledge of the common and less common adverse outcomes of minor surgery to the skin.
- Carry out a significant event audit for a minor surgery procedure that has had an adverse outcome involving you and the practice nurse.
- Design a simple patient questionnaire to establish whether patients have understood your explanations of the advantages and disadvantages of having a minor surgical procedure performed. Compare the patients' understanding with the information you intended to communicate to them.

Stage 3B: Identify your service needs

> Any of the needs assessment exercises in 3A may also reveal service needs.

- Check that up-to-date consent forms are readily available at your practice for any minor surgery procedure.
- Interview individual staff in the practice to identify any potential failings in the system used in your practice to ensure that informed written consent is given prior to minor surgical procedures or similar activities (such as fitting intra-uterine coils).
- Undertake an audit of the last 25 patients who have had minor surgery performed in the practice. Establish for what percentage there are consent forms on file, and how many were correctly completed.

Stage 4: Make and carry out a learning and action plan

- Undertake an informal visit to a minor surgery clinic in another practice or local hospital.
- Attend a formal minor surgery course.
- Download and study a copy of Consent Form 3 from the Department of Health's consent pages at: www.dh.gov.uk/assetRoot/04/07/46/57/04074657.rtf.
- Arrange an educational in-house meeting for those members of your primary care team involved in minor surgery. Topics covered will include the importance of obtaining valid informed consent as well as practical techniques, sterilisation of equipment, etc.

Stage 5: Document your learning, competence, performance and standards of service delivery

- Collect and keep the documentation relating to the processes outlined in Stages 3 and 4 above.
- Repeat the audits and patient questionnaires to monitor the effects of changes on standards achieved relating to informed consent.
- Record the significant event audit and the subsequent analysis of events. Add your notes about subsequent changes in practice and any re-audit.
- Keep a copy of the informed consent form for minor surgery plus other versions for different purposes.

Case study 10.5 continued

You explain that clinically both of the moles appear to be benign. You discuss the procedures necessary to remove these lesions as well as the potential risks involved with minor surgery. You are sufficiently concerned about the risk of keloid scar formation at the shoulder tip site that you state that you would not operate for a clinically benign lesion without very good reason. You offer to remove the pedunculated papule on the lateral thorax by shave excision and suggest a policy of monitoring regarding the pigmented naevus on the shoulder. Ms Mole agrees to this plan.

Two weeks later she attends your minor surgery clinic. You again explain the nature and intended benefits as well as the serious or frequently occurring risks of the procedure. You discuss the alternatives to surgery. These include doing nothing. Ms Mole still wishes you to proceed with surgery. You complete Consent Form 3 together, which she then signs. The procedure itself is uneventful.

On review six weeks later the wound has healed well. Histology confirms a benign intradermal naevus. Ms Mole is happy with the outcome of her surgery.

References

1 www.medicines-partnership.org/about-us/concordance

2 Joint Formulary Committee (2004) *British National Formulary. BNF 47*. British Medical Association and Royal Pharmaceutical Society of Great Britain, London.

3 Gawkrodger DJ (1997) *Dermatology an Illustrated Colour Text* (2e). Churchill Livingstone, Edinburgh.

4 www.eczema.org

5 General Practitioners Committee/The NHS Confederation (2003) *New GMS Contract. Investing in general practice*. General Practitioners Committee/NHS Confederation, London.

Further resources

Patient support groups

- National Eczema Society, Hill House, Highgate Hill, London N19 5NA, UK. Office tel: +44 (0)20 7281 3553; fax: +44 (0)20 7281 6395; telephone helpline: +44 (0)870 241 3604 (8am to 8pm Monday to Friday). www.eczema.org
- Psoriasis Association (UK): www.psoriasis-association.org.uk
- Raynaud's and Scleroderma Association, 112 Crewe Road, Alsager, Cheshire ST7 2JA, UK. Tel: +44 (0)1270 872776; fax: +44 01270 883556; email: info@raynauds.org.uk; www.raynauds.org.uk/flash_content.html

Societies

- For more in-depth dermatological studies: DermIS main menu. Includes an online dermatological atlas: www.dermis.net/index_e.htm
- Primary Care Dermatology Society. A national society for GPs with a special interest in dermatology: www.pcds.org.uk
- Information on the British Society of Dermatological Surgery: www. bad.org.uk
- Information on the Diploma in Practical Dermatology run by the Department of Dermatology, University of Wales College of Medicine: www.ukdermatology. co.uk/asp/dpd.asp

And finally

We hope that you have found that the stages in our 'cycle of evidence' are a useful approach to gathering information about what you need to learn. You can also use it to identify improvements you or others need to make to the way you deliver services.

It is easy to feel overwhelmed by the magnitude of the task to demonstrate that you are competent and perform consistently well as a doctor, in order to retain your licence to practise. Remember that you should be producing evidence about the breadth of your practice, every five years. Take your time and select three or four cycles of evidence each year that span several headings of *Good Medical Practice* at one time.[1]

Ask others for help. Your practice manager or the receptionists should be able to help you to collect information about what you need to learn, or about gaps in services. You can delegate much of the administrative side. Your colleagues or your patients will be well placed to help you to set your aspirations for good practice and set achievable standards for your outcomes – of learning and improvements in service delivery. Perhaps your CPD tutor can help you to develop learning and action in your PDP. These cycles of evidence will be the nucleus of your PDP. Colleagues in the team can support you in documenting the evidence of your competence, performance and subsequent standards of service delivery. Other books in this series might help you to look at specific clinical areas, especially those where quality frameworks or special interests require your attention. Remember to visit the book's supporting website, which includes useful website links.[2]

So the evidence will be there ready to submit for appraisal interviews or revalidation, but the results will show what a good doctor you really are. This should give you increasing confidence and self-respect. Enjoy your professional glow.

References

1 General Medical Council (2001) *Good Medical Practice*. General Medical Council, London.

2 http://health.mattersonline.net

Index